# The Principles and Practice of
# Clinical Trials

# The Principles and Practice of Clinical Trials

*Based on a Symposium organised by the*
*Association of Medical Advisers in the*
*Pharmaceutical Industry*

Edited by

C.S. GOOD, M.A., B.M., B.Ch., F.R.C.S.
Senior Medical Adviser, Bayer U.K. Limited,
Pharmaceuticals Division

Foreword by

SIR CYRIL CLARKE, K.B.E., M.D., P.R.C.P., F.R.S.
President of the Royal College of Physicians, London

CHURCHILL LIVINGSTONE
EDINBURGH LONDON AND NEW YORK
1976

CHURCHILL LIVINGSTONE
Medical Division of Longman Group Limited


Distributed in the United States of America by
Longman Inc., 19 West 44th Street, New York,
N.Y. 10036 and by associated companies,
branches and representatives throughout
the world.

ISBN 0 443 01525 2

Printed in Great Britain by
T. & A. Constable Ltd., Edinburgh

# Foreword

The medical and pharmaceutical professions have a responsibility not only for the prevention of disease and the cure of the sick but also for the advancement of knowledge. Here clinical trials of drugs play an important part.

In 1969 the Association of Medical Advisers in the Pharmaceutical Industry organised a symposium held in the Royal College of Physicians of London on the principles and practice of such trials. My predecessor, Lord Rosenheim, wrote the foreword to the book which followed. It reflected the happy state of affairs at the time and it seemed then that the barometer was set fair for mutual cooperation and progress. It is true that there have been great therapeutic advances in the intervening years; but increasing knowledge of the complexity of drugs and of their interactions, and more appreciation of the ethical problems involved, made it seem appropriate to have a second conference. Therefore, as President of the Royal College of Physicians, I was delighted when the Association of Medical Advisers in the Pharmaceutical Industry decided to do so.

The title of the 1976 symposium remains the same and the book reporting it contains much new and valuable information. The chapter headings show the variety of the topics discussed and in general there is a more critical attitude than in 1969. The essence, however, remains the same and can be distilled, as Dr. Burley points out in simple words from the Old Testament:

How long halt ye between two opinions? If The Lord be God, follow him: but if Baal, then follow him.

CYRIL A. CLARKE

June 1976

# Preface

This book is intended for use by medical advisers in the pharmaceutical industry and clinicians who are involved in the evaluation of drugs. It is designed mainly for those new to the field, as was the first edition, but it also contains much useful information for those with experience who wish to improve their knowledge or expand their interest. The highly successful first edition went out of print last year. Many aspects had changed since it was published. Therefore a fresh symposium with the same title was held again at the Royal College of Physicians, on the 6th and 7th May 1976, to bring the material up to date.

This book is based on papers presented at that symposium, and this time it includes the recorded discussions. These help to highlight some of the problems not covered or clarified in the papers. The further developments in clinical trials to which this book pays particular attention are: the rapidly increasing costs of trials, and how to budget for them; the increasing complexity of statutory regulations; the somewhat arbitrary division of clinical trials into Phases I to IV; the great increase in attempts to monitor adverse reactions and the development of drug surveillance programmes; the advances in data handling and statistical analysis.

As with the first edition, the book is laid out according to the development of a clinical trial. It ends with five common areas for drug evaluation, which are examples of the principles laid down in the first part. There is a comprehensive list of references for further reading at the end of most chapters.

I wish to thank all the chairmen and contributors for their willing help and understanding; the section organisers Dr. M.J. Boyce, Dr. R.B. Khambatta, Dr. B.T. Marsh and Dr. M.J. Tidd who offered their unstinting help in organising the symposium; Mrs. J. Wase-Bailey who was responsible for all the administration; the Trust for Education and Research in Therapeutics for the idea and advice; the Royal College of Physicians for help and hospitality; the publishers, Churchill Livingstone, for guidance and assistance in getting the book published; Mrs. G. Feltham for coping with the indecipherable discussions; and all those without whose help it would not have been possible, in particular my long-suffering wife.

1976                                                                          C.S. GOOD

vii

# Chairmen

Sir Cyril Clarke, KBE, MD, PRCP, FRS. President of the Royal College of Physicians, London.

Dr. G. Beaumont, MB, ChB, DObst RCOG, DCH. Chairman of AMAPI and Medical Adviser, Geigy Pharmaceuticals, Macclesfield.

Professor T.D.V. Lawrie, MD, FRCP (Edin. & Glas.) Walton Professor of Medical Cardiology, Royal Infirmary, Glasgow.

Dr. P.A. Nicholson, MB, BS. Medical Director, Hoechst U.K. Limited, Pharmaceutical Division, Hounslow.

# List of Contributors

G. Beaumont, MB, ChB, DObst RCOG, DCH. Medical Department, Geigy Pharmaceuticals, Macclesfield.

D.M. Burley, MB, BS, MRCS, LRCP. Head of Medical Services, CIBA Laboratories, Horsham.

P.G.T. Bye, BA, MB, BChir, DCH. Senior Medical Adviser, Schering Chemicals Limited, Burgess Hill.

M.F. Cuthbert, MB, BS, PhD. Principal Medical Officer, Medicines Division, Department of Health and Social Security, London.

A.W. Galbraith, MA, MB, BChir, DObst RCOG, DCH. General Practitioner, 26 Abercorn Place, London.

F. Grady, Data Services Section, Imperial Chemical Industries Limited, Macclesfield.

J.J. Grimshaw, BSc, FIS. Consultant Statistician, Wessex Consultancy, Aldershot.

A.W. Harcus, MB, ChB, DObst RCOG. Medical Director, Reckitt and Colman, Kingston-upon-Hull.

C.F. Hawkins, MD, FRCP. Consultant Physician to the Central Birmingham Health District. The Queen Elizabeth Hospital, Birmingham.

W.S. Hillis, MB, MRCP (U.K.) Senior Registrar in Cardiology, University Department of Medical Cardiology, Royal Infirmary, Glasgow.

E.C. Huskisson, MD, MRCP. Consultant Physician, St. Leonard's Hospital, London, and Senior Lecturer in the Medical College of St. Bartholomew's Hospital, London.

I.M. James, MRCP, MB, BS, PhD. Senior Lecturer in Medicine and Therapeutics, Medical Unit, The Royal Free Hospital, London.

T.D.V. Lawrie, MD, FRCP (Edin. & Glas.) Walton Professor of Medical Cardiology, Royal Infirmary, Glasgow.

K.D. MacRae, MA, PhD. Senior Lecturer in Statistics, Charing Cross Hospital Medical School, London.

B.T. Marsh, MB, BS (Hnrs.) DObst RCOG. Medical Director, Leo Laboratories Limited, Hayes, Middlesex.

P.A. Nicholson, MB, BS. Medical Director, Hoechst U.K. Limited, Pharmaceutical Division, Hounslow.

D.S. Reeves, MB, MRCPath. Consultant Medical Microbiologist, Department of Medical Microbiology, Southmead General Hospital, Bristol.

R.B. Smith, BSc, MD. Research and Development Director, Reckitt and Colman, Kingston-upon-Hull.

E.S. Snell, MA, MD, FRCP. Director, Clinical Division, Glaxo Research Limited, Greenford.

A.C. Tweddel, MB, ChB. Registrar in Cardiology, University Department of Medical Cardiology, Royal Infirmary, Glasgow.

D.W. Vere, MD, FRCP. Professor of Therapeutics at The London Hospital Medical College, University of London.

# Contents

# PART 1
# SETTING UP CLINICAL TRIALS

# 1. Ethics of Clinical Trials

D. W. VERE

Medicine is an interference with persons. It is tolerated and supported only because the overwhelming balance of its effects is expected to be in patients' interests to bring them benefit rather than harm. The public tolerates Medicine only when all reasonable steps are seen to have been taken to guarantee benefit with safety. Some demand complete safety; more informed patients are prepared to accept that accidental or unforeseeable hurts can happen and indeed must be expected at times just as they occur in the rest of life. Ethics are a rational analysis of moral behaviour, that is of that part of behaviour which happens when people feel they ought to do something. With clinical trials, ethics are largely concerned with four things: the defeat of disease, the safety of subjects, the conservation of natural resources and the sharing of knowledge. Our duty to do what is good and right exceeds these four. This includes protection in industry, in warfare, in sport and in travel. There are different views about how we learn what is right, but there is a wide area over which most people can reach practical agreement.

Thurston (1966) expressed the ethical onus in a nutshell, 'Do nothing which would undermine trust'. Perhaps one should add to that, 'in any rational, informed and disinterested person'. How can this aim be achieved and safeguarded? Some would say by codes, and there are many codes. Codes have a proper place in stating important generalities, but are restrictive and legalistic if pressed to detail.

Bradford Hill (1963) proposed that the detailed problems are better dealt with by asking questions than by applying codes. He had a check-list of questions for intending investigators to apply to their proposed trials. His judgement still seems to have been entirely right. No attempt will be made to review the history of ethical proposals in this chapter, but rather to see what extensions might be made to Bradford Hill's check-list after thirteen years. His check-list included these headings:

1. Is the proposed treatment safe........is it unlikely to do harm to the patient?

2. Can a new treatment ethically be withheld from any patients in the doctor's care?

3. What patients may be brought into a controlled trial and allocated randomly to different treatments?

4. Is it necessary to obtain the patient's consent to his inclusion in a controlled trial?

5. Is it ethical to use a placebo, or dummy treatment?

6. Is it proper for the doctor not to know the treatment being administered to his patient?

3

Clinical trials are acceptable only as a part of medicine. They have no other primary justification, be it social, commercial, scientific or political. This is not to deny that scientific, commercial or other interests may also be satisfied when there is a proper medical reason for making a trial. Trials in general are acceptable only as an essential part of making sick people better; any proposed exception to this general rule must be scrutinised most critically.

The primary ethical reasons for making trials were stated with persuasive and admirable clarity by Bradford Hill. Better treatments are needed. To find a better treatment one must make a comparison. The most reliable method for making comparisons is the scientific method, which is more reliable than personal experience and which tackles the problem of bias. An acceptable pattern of ethical decision emerges:

Better treatments are needed

They are best chosen by scientific comparison.

Comparative, 'controlled' trials are justified only when it is uncertain which of two remedies is the better; and it is likely that a new remedy is at least as good as, or better than, the established treatment.

If that is agreed, many provocative exceptions to the pattern appear, particularly as a result of recent drug developments. I will discuss these without being too specific about the meaning of 'trial'. I will include all stages of drug testing in man, whether new remedies or new indications, and attend to present rather than past problems.

The problems may be divided conveniently into those of the general aims and objectives of trials, those of the recruitment of subjects, those of the conduct of trials, those involving outside agencies (ethics committees, regulatory bodies, insurers) and those of the effects of trials on Medicine as a whole.

## Aims and objectives of trials

Everyone knows the first ethical difficulty. No-one can do much about it at present, but it is worth remembering in case it may become soluble. In an ideal world drugs would be designed to combat specific diseases. Most attempts to do this have failed, and it would be a costly way to innovate until we really know the mechanisms of disease. Meanwhile there are industrial reasons for a company to exploit one chemical structure and its derivatives for which they have patent protection, working them out as miners exhaust a seam of coal. Most people settle for the common approach and synthesise numbers of new compounds, screening them in a search for possible remedies with any useful actions. One result has been the discovery of a handful of really important and surprising drugs. Another is the production of scores of drugs with closely similar actions - anticholinergics, anti-inflammatory or antihistamine drugs - none of which has more than the slenderest advantage over any other. Charity might class this activity as a necessary evil, but other terms are being introduced to describe the more wasteful aspects of this massive use of resources. It would be easier to accept if, as when one pans for gold, the gravel could be discarded. But often the brighter bits of gravel in this enterprise are sold as gold.

It is difficult to adapt to the changing world. In a sense it is not the world that changes but our view of it. Yesterday it was vast and unexplored, waiting to be exploited. Today it is of finite size, to be conserved: We are learning to join in with its recyclings rather than to distort or defeat them. There is no shortage of chemical ingenuity. But there are marked shortages of some natural resource like available energy, and human resources like volunteer subjects for trials and skilled staff. It therefore seems essential to stop and think again before deciding, for example, to develop another beta blocker or analgesic for commercial reasons (such as balancing a company's product profile) rather than because there is human need. Against this there is always the occasionally justified argument that a dull but lucrative compound may turn up novel and useful properties.

Must all trials aim to benefit patients directly? (Royal College of Physicians, 1973; Bradford Hill, 1963). The answer to this question may at first seem obvious, but it runs away from you as you pursue it. All trials involve a balance of profit and loss to the subjects. The profits may include occasionally the discovery of a better remedy for them. At least they usually get a good medical check from the procedure. But the gains may be collective rather than individual, and future rather than present, for others not for self. The losses, off work, time, travel, prescription charges, and the risks of adverse and often unexpected effects of novel drugs are almost always trivial but can be irritating. The subjects of trials give much altruism and unselfish care. It is essential not to exploit this scarce human resource.

Should a new treatment be expected to be better than, or as good as, existing treatments before it is put to trial? Again, the answer seems obvious until it is closely examined. Bradford Hill repeatedly implied that it was proper to bring a remedy to trial if it appeared likely to confer benefit with safety. But events during these thirteen years make it necessary to look afresh at these problems. Two events in particular, the appearance of prodigious numbers of alternative remedies, and the disaster of delayed adverse reactions, give one pause. Manufacturers are now in a position to develop tens or scores of derivatives of the same chemical nucleus, yielding whole families of roughly equivalent drugs. Examples are the arylaliphatic acid anti-inflammatory drugs, and the many series of compounds which in general have properties very like the tricyclic antidepressants. Examples of late, unpredictable and sometimes horrible adverse effects are methyldopa, practolol and aminorex. Any one of all these compounds seems, at the time it is brought to trial, likely to confer benefit with safety. But it is a dubious ethical use of precious volunteers and natural resources to test a score of drugs when only one is needed and only short term safety and efficacy can be explored. The benefits gained are probably not even commensurate with the losses. The impasse is that any one of these trials may be ethical, but that a hundred of them may not be.

A few manufacturers bring compounds of undistinguished efficacy and dubious toxicity again and again before regulatory bodies. It is easy to see the commercial reasons for this, but is it ethically justifiable? A new criterion is needed, which is horribly difficult to envisage or apply. Superiority over existing remedies or a novel mode of action is needed beyond probable 'benefit with safety', for a compound to gain acceptance in terms of public need. At present there seems to be no fair, practical and right solution to this problem. It is a major ethical issue of today, and must be faced. It is a poor thing if medical gain is reduced to a trivial pretext of commerce; if drugs which are likely to be worse than others are tested in case they may be better; if people get starry-eyed about their potential products. But, if one has lived with and dreamed of a promising new compound for some years it is difficult to see it die.

There is a point which is widely known and ignored. The criterion of trial success is taken as statistical significance. But mere statistical significance is not enough; the result should be a biological and economic success if the drug is to stand the test of ethical worth. We may now need to add another question to Bradford Hill's checklist, 'Is this trial likely to yield information of novel and real clinical benefit?' The answer with some drugs that are at present at this stage of development can only be 'no'.

It will at once be argued that manufacturers are not prophets; no-one can foresee which drug may prove to be a 'winner', and those who pay the staggering cost of developing a compound to the trial stage deserve a fair return for their efforts. Otherwise they cannot even remain in business. Against this, we must ask whether the public should be asked to pay for the losses in money, or by eating larger quantities of potentially toxic and scarcely appropriate tablets, or both? There is at present no real solution to this dilemma, but sooner or later the public will want to take more part in the choice. This has great risks, for public pressure usually takes the form of more control by bureaux. Modell (1976) has written that though we aim to have progress with safety, the only way to safety is through progress. We learn best to avoid disasters by having them. It is not wrong to have a disaster; it is disastrously wrong to fail to try to avoid it, and to fail to make the maximum use of the information which can be learned from it. There cannot be drugs without some personal injuries; but it is as wrong to court disaster by halting progress as it is by multiplying unnecessary drugs. The ethically acceptable course is for all to search together for the best 'critical path' through the maze of biochemical innovation. This path will not be found by 'adversary groups' who press opposing views to deadlock.

This leads to the most subtle ethical problem of all, the problem of prime motivation. Two companies may aim to develop drugs. One does it primarily with an altruistic aim, to defeat disease, to promote health. The other does it with a primarily commercial aim, to make money, to gain power or prestige. Both may develop the same compound and ask for clinical help with identical trials. It does not matter chemically, scientifically or medically what their motives are. But it does matter crucially to every patient who is given the drug. The difference in motive begins to show at once in the care that is taken of people.

Most trials lie between these two extremes; they have both medical and commercial interests, usually of a wholly proper kind (ABPI Report, Section 3.1). The problem is that the commercial interest so easily displaces the medical interest. Which gains the upper hand when there is a difficult ethical decision about patient care? That is the acid test. Again, Bradford Hill was right. There is no code, no rule, no law which can get it right. Where rules fail, personal encounter succeeds. A clinical investigator who meets industry closely at a personal level can soon diagnose where a company's prime motive lies. The ethical safeguard is to decline to work with people who do not keep high standards of subject care. But there is still a problem. There are clinical investigators who keep poor standards. In Europe in recent years, there have been trials made without the subjects' knowledge and informed consent, some in mentally sick patients of drugs for cardiovascular disorders, some in peasants who would neither know nor care if an explanation were offered them. It is therefore sometimes not enough to trust the ethical sense of clinicians or companies.

How should firms relate to clinical trialists? Some have suggested setting up units, specifically for the conduct of trials (Parkhouse, 1966; Uvarov, 1967) so that the industry would not have to go 'cap in hand to the medical profession to get worthwhile compounds tested'. Unhappily the industry and the profession may not always agree about what is a 'worthwhile compound' and Laurence (1964) had a wiser emphasis when he commented that 'there is seldom any difficulty with new compounds of obvious theoretical or particular practical interest'.

One last problem needs airing in this general section. When is a trial a survey, and how far should industrial surveys go? It is a necessary part of industrial organisation to get information about product use, both one's own product and one's competitors'. Extensive market research operations are undertaken, some with the apparent purpose of conditioning prescribers and often through intermediaries who do not disclose their customers' identity. That is outside the scope of this chapter. However, a half way house is beginning to appear, linked with the so called 'general practitioner trial'. Suppose that company X empanels a very large number of general practitioners, and invites them to report to the company their experiences with Y patients given Z drugs, including perhaps one of X's products. Now, with *small* values for Y and Z this is a type of open trial. With very large numbers of Y and Z what is it? It is no longer a statistically valid exercise, because with large numbers statistical significance becomes biologically meaningless. It is not market research, for the doctors may not always have made their usual, spontaneous prescribing choices.

It tends towards market research, however, and poses many problems. What would happen if every company started to do this? To whom would the information belong? Would it be published? It could not be published in the scientific literature, for it is not scientific. Could prescribing choice eventually be conditioned by industry, if many prescriptions were part of such 'trials'? This is like *1984*, but we do have only eight years to start thinking. Any firm which mounts surveys of this kind carries a heavy burden of public accountability.

## Trial subjects

The next set of problems concerns trial subjects. Three are prominent: 'informed consent', trials in those who cannot consent, and payment to volunteers.

The 'informed consent' problem is much debated (Bradford Hill, 1963; ABPI Report). Bradford Hill listed several situations where consent need *not* be solicited. There is no general solution, but a few ideas may be useful. The members of the department in which I work have been impressed by two ideas; that most 'lay' volunteers can not be informed in any meaningful sense, and that it is helpful to have a 'subject's friend'. Volunteers can not be informed because they have no technical expertise. They are therefore able neither to understand technical information, nor to make use of it even when put in their own language. If you tell a volunteer in east London that there is a remote statistical probability that a fatality could occur he will not understand you; if you tell him in his own terms that 'there's outside odds that it might knock yer off' he will either conclude quite wrongly that there is no gain for him and leave, or equally wrongly may volunteer smilingly, saying, 'Well, I have to leave all that to you, doc'. We try to conduct volunteer interviews using an extension of the 'patients's friend' idea. When a volunteer comes to interview we ask a graduate from another department, in no way beholden to us, to come to the meeting. He is asked to put himself entirely on the subject's side, to listen to the explanation, to ask questions about it in the subject's presence, and to satisfy himself that a meaningful, sufficient explanation of the risks and benefits has been given and that the subject understood it. He then signs the form to say that he witnessed the subject's verbal consent, and that in his opinion a satisfactory explanation was given and understood. For volunteers there may be no such thing as 'informed consent', but there can be 'safeguarded consent'.

Another problem surrounds those who *cannot* consent, children, the very aged, mental patients and the unconscious. A difference of view about trials on children has arisen between the legal profession (and those official medical bodies who follow their judgements) and the Royal College of Physicians. It seems odd if ethical safeguards cannot be agreed for trials of drugs which sick children need, after testing in adults. The obstacles at present are: Legal precedent; the legal inability of parents to consent; the public outcry if something does go wrong in a trial on children; reliance on codes rather than on honest questions about the ethics of a trial. Children are probably suffering at present because certain researches cannot be made into their complaints. Some excellent and entirely helpful trials have been made by unofficial bodies. One remarkable example (Valentine and Maxwell, 1968) was made in mentally retarded children by an employee of a drug firm and a hospital superintendent and showed successfully that a treatment used as a routine for enuresis was quite ineffective, though human care and attention could succeed. Could anything be more ethically satisfying than that? I believe that nothing would be more disastrous than an attempt to regulate this matter by more detailed legislation. We need an ethical scheme to ensure that the right questions are asked, the best safeguards applied, and that there are some guarded exceptions to the ban on parental consent. This scheme could be better achieved by the Royal Colleges and the industry's associations working together than by legislation.

Payments to subjects or investigators are emotive, because people fail to distinguish between indulgent payment to secure collaboration on one hand, and normal fees (agreed by a professional association) or reimbursements for time used on the other. The former are distasteful, open to abuse, and attractive to criticism. The latter are proper. Those who make proper payments of the latter kind should say so publicly; they have no need to feel ashamed. Why should those making proper trials suffer financially as well as give their time? There is a social duty to participate in trials, and reimbursement is just for those who do. But payment as a financial inducement to make promotional trials is odious.

In the trial itself there are problems about placebos, and about statistical advice. Some people think that placebos are inactive remedies, and so deceive patients in an unethical way. This is certainly not so; placebos are not totally inactive, they are pharmacologically inactive. Lasagna, Laties and Dihan (1958) have produced ample evidence that they produce effects, and that these effects have a time course of action resembling that of pharmacologically active agents. We have confirmed this repeatedly to incredulous classes of medical students. So has Blackwell *et al.* (1972). It is not the case that drugs confer benefit while placebos do not. A drug is only more than a placebo if it confers *more* benefit than a placebo. There need be no ethical problem. Patients can be told in all honesty that they will be given each of a pair of drugs at different times, both likely to be beneficial, but acting in different ways, one through its effects on the mind, the other partly like that and also partly affecting the body. If they are told that they are to receive 'an inactive treatment' they may feel justifiably upset. It is possible that placebos only simulate expected benefits but do not confer any physical relief from physical disorders. They may only affect what the subject experiences, not what he physically is, and so are in a sense a more cruel cheat than if they conferred no apparent benefits at all. This theory cannot be tested at present, but will ensure that the debate goes on.

Statistical advice during a trial is fraught with difficulty, ethical and statistical. In a double blind trial, how does a physician know when to stop? We have known cases where patients who suffered an 'adverse reaction' were in the placebo group, and others where real drug damage became apparent to the statistical workers who knew the code, but was missed by physicians who did not. Our answer, no doubt imperfect, is to involve the statistician in the trial as a 'controller'. He is not a mere code holder. He relates the code to the clinical records without informing the trial physicians, and 'trouble shoots' as the trial goes on. If he notices a systematic adverse effect he inter-venes in the patients' interest and may stop part or all of the trial. There is a lot of importance in the word 'notices', because a statistician might not notice anything that had not reached significance. The controller must analyse the trial progressively as it goes along, by appropriate methods. Should he intervene in a block trial when it reaches sequential significance with respect to the benefits rather than the adverse effects of the test drug? The answer is that as a rule he should not intervene, for several reasons: block designs are unstructured with respect to time, sequential designs are structured; block size is decided beforehand on the available criteria to give the most valid statistical probabilities; sequential design is prepared for economy with pre-fixed probabilities. But he *should* intervene for reasons of safety. We therefore always have a 'trial controller', or perhaps 'trial coordinator' might be a better name. Bradford Hill criticised the statistician who sat at an Olympian distance from the trial and urged that he should involve himself directly as part of the team. We have tried to elaborate his good advice.

There are many cases of bias introduced into trial comparisons. These are so evi-dently wrong, on both ethical and scientific grounds, that there is no need to discuss them further.

### Regulatory bodies, and other external influences on trials

These authorities are another necessary evil, but need not be quite so evil as they are at times. They are the law, the ethics committees, the Committee on Safety of Medicines and the insurers. The law can indeed be 'an ass', since it cannot always control its ruthless logic so as to promote what is good. A distinguished lawyer has said that all clinical trials are at legal risk because they may involve withdrawing a remedy of proven efficacy, replacing it by one which *may* be ineffective. This opinion may be excellent law, but it is scientific and social nonsense. Not only is there always some doubt about the efficacy of the existing remedy, but it is also true that there would be no existing remedies had they not been shown, often by trials, to be superior to others. If to fulfil the law means to abolish advance in medicine, it seems likely that the public will ignore the law and prefer progress. The law seems to be calculatedly unhelpful in most matters of medical progress, and the clinical trial is no exception (Mugglestone, 1975). If only there were a disease peculiar to lawyers for which a cure could only be established by clinical trial!

Ethics committees, though necessary, can be tiresome. They seem unable to decide why they exist; to protect subjects, to protect investigators, to make that which is emotionally unacceptable to some people seem respectable, to give advice on ethical problems, to assess the scientific and ethical nature of proposals? Some force badly worded consent forms upon hapless investigators. One form insisted that every trialist must get his patients to sign their agreement to his doing what he was not in fact about to do! It made the patient say that he recognised that any treatments he might receive might not be part of his necessary treatment, which of course is exactly what a good trial is not. So, in effect, it made every patient agree that his physician was about to do a bad trial, and the physician had to witness it by his own signature!

Large numbers of detailed ethical problems arise over national regulation of drug safety. The two mentioned here are among the effects of having any regulations, rather than effects directly imposed by the regulatory authority. First, in an attempt to get a drug past the regulatory authority, many companies set up numerous trials with small numbers of patients, when large numbers may be needed to study patients' acceptance of a remedy. Adverse reactions are too rare to be noticed in most of these trials, which therefore tend to amplify the advantages over the disadvantages of a new drug. These points outlined by Bradford Hill towards the end of the first section of his check-list, but even he may not have foreseen the size that this problem would assume. It seems right that companies should follow their initial trials with surveys of their product to go some way to meet this need.

The second problem is that the value of the formal process of regulation is diluted progressively as more and more compounds are thrust upon it. It may be possible to evade the system by saturating it, and the immense productivity of industry may at times achieve this.

But, as we have seen, this flood of innovation is not really one of new ideas and drug effects. It is a flood of whole classes of similar compounds.

A problem which is perhaps more practical than ethical is that there is no satis-factory insurance available against non-negligent injury during trials. It would be difficult enough to arrange this for volunteer studies, but quite impossible to imagine how to achieve it for clinical trials.

Over all these problems there is the question which uniquely troubles regulatory bodies: Are trials regarded as a mere extension of toxicology to man, as the final member of a team of 'animals' needed to provide enough evidence to pass the regulatory body? If trials are refused in one country, should they then be done in another which protects its citizens less well, and the results then used to pass the barriers in the first country? Bradford Hill faced this honestly, insisting that 'human experiment' is the only way to gain beneficial knowledge. But the ABPI report on experiments on staff volunteers asserts that, 'studies of drugs in volunteers cannot be justified as a mere extension of toxicity tests on experimental animals'. The difference cited in that report between animal tests and human volunteer studies is simply that the human tests are to be preceded by animal studies made in species which handle the new drug in a manner similar to man. How do you detect that similarity without first making some experi-ments in man? The real difference between animal and human tests is that animals are given large doses, whereas man is given gradually increasing doses, so that risks can be confined to as few people as possible and the extent of damage minimised. Some reports do not show that this cautious, gradual approach was used, but merely list the results of tests in a number of persons. It would halp if regulatory bodies insisted upon a description of the way in which these data were obtained, even if the subjects came from other nations.

### The impact on medicine as a whole

Lastly, what of the effects of the whole system for testing new drugs upon Medicine? It is true that new and worthwhile drugs have been developed by the pharmaceutical industry. It is also true that trials are encouraging a more scientific approach to therapy. I suspect that it is also true that the prolific efforts of that industry are conditioning us all to believe that the main answers to medical problems are drugs, that we should constantly look to new drugs to transcend the old, and that the advertiser's choice should be the prescriber's choice. We are constantly pressed to believe that in trial work statistical significance is the end point, when it is biological significance that really matters. None of these adverse attitudes benefits the nation's health; we should culti-vate a searchingly critical attitude towards them. Some trials are contrived as costly and elaborate confidence tricks, and unjustified claims built upon them. Others are excellent pieces of scientific work, among the best to hand.

In summary, my suggested additions to Bradford Hill's remarkably prescient check-list would be:

1. How should consent be obtained?

2. Even if all statutory requirements are satisfied, is a trial justified biologically, or by human need? Is this compound going to trial primarily for its medical promise, or primarily for commercial reasons?

3. Who should be told the results of trial work, and how?

4. Should there be a 'trial controller', or 'coordinator', and how should he relate to the clinicians?

These are only extensions of what Bradford Hill said; they are all present in germ at least amongst his ideas, but they need to be spelt out with increasing clarity as the problems grow more sophisticated and far reaching in their effects.

The only way to safeguard a satisfactory ethical structure for clinical trials is to keep the decisions in the hands of an independent medical profession which is working for the patients' and subjects' interests. But if any part of the ethical structure becomes a 'private garden' of a group of doctors, politicians, lawyers, industrialists or any combination of these, then there are enormous dangers to trial subjects and to Medicine.

It is a pleasure to acknowledge the help of Dr. T.B. Binns who kindly read and comm-ented on this paper. Though the views expressed are not necessarily his, the rare moments of clarity owe much to his careful help.

REFERENCES

A.B.P.I. Report, 'The report of the committee to investigate medical experiments on staff volunteers'. Section 3.1. Issued by the Association of the British Pharmaceutical Industry, London.

Blackwell, B., Bloomfield, S.S. & Buncher, C.R. (1972) Demonstration to medical students of placebo-responses and non-drug factors. *Lancet,* 10th June, 1279.

Bradford Hill, Sir A.(1963) Medical ethics and controlled trials. *British Medical Journal,* 20th April, 1043 - 1049.

Lasagna, L., Laties, V.G. & Dihan, J.L. (1958) Further studies on the pharmacology of placebo administration. *Journal of Clinical Investigation,* **37**, 533 - 537.

Laurence, D.R. (1964) Clinical Pharmacology. *Lancet,* **1**,1173.

Modell, W. (1976) Progress with protection. *Clinical Pharmacology and Therapeutics,* **19**, 121 - 123.

Mugglestone, C.J. (1975) Safeguards for healthy volunteers in drug studies. *Lancet,* 22nd November, 1047.

Parkhouse, J. (1966) Some thoughts on the clinical evaluation of drugs. *Postgraduate Medical Journal,* **42**, 748.

Royal College of Physicians (1973) Supervision of ethics of clinical research investigations in institutions, *Royal College of Physicians,* 2b.

Royal College of Physicians (1974) President's Annual Address, *Royal College of Physicians,* 6.

Thurston, G. (1966) Problems of consent. *British Medical Journal,* 1405 - 1407.

Uvarov, O. (1968) Clinical evaluation of drugs in man and animals. *Proceedings of the Royal Society of Medicine,* **61**, 569 - 574.

Valentine, A.A. & Maxwell, C. (1968) Enuresis in severely subnormal children - a clinical trial of impramine. *Journal of Mental Subnormality,* **14**, Part 2.

# 2. Regulations Relating to Clinical Trials

M. F. CUTHBERT

Despite high standards which generally existed in the pharmaceutical industry, until 1964 there was no necessity for a manufacturer to seek approval from an independent body before commencing clinical trials or putting a new drug on the market. These matters did not come under control until the Committee on Safety of Drugs was established in January 1964 in consultation with the medical and pharmaceutical professions and with the pharmaceutical industry following the thalidomide disaster. Although the terms of reference of the Committee were to review the available evidence for new drugs and to advise on their toxicity, the Committee had no legal powers and operated strictly on a voluntary basis. A very important consideration to the successful operation of this system was that the major pharmaceutical manufacturers (members of the Proprietary Association of Great Britain and of the Association of the British Pharmaceutical Industry) agreed to seek the Committee's approval before commencing clinical trials with a new drug and also before placing it on the market. The voluntary system worked well but it was realised that this was only an interim measure until comprehensive legislation could be established to provide legal controls over the sale and supply of medicines.

## Medicines Act (1968)

The Medicines Act (1968) is a comprehensive piece of legislation. It was implemented in September 1971 and exercises control over the manufacturing, importation, sale and supply, labelling and advertising of medicines. A Medicines Commission has been established to give general advice on the various aspects of the enforcement of the Act. It also functions as an appeal body in respect of the activities of a number of expert advisory committees. In the context of this chapter the most relevant of these expert committees is the Committee on Safety of Medicines which has replaced the Committee on Safety of Drugs. The Committee on Safety of Medicines is served by a number of expert sub-committees and advises on the issuing of licences and certificates. The Licensing Authority issues Clinical Trial Certificates, valid for two years, for drugs approved by the Committee on Safety of Medicines; and Product Licences, valid for five years, for drugs similarly approved for marketing.

Before a clinical trial can be conducted on a new drug in the United Kingdom, the supplier must hold a valid Clinical Trial Certificate. It should be emphasised that the Act does not prohibit the carrying out of trials which have not been authorised; what it does do is to prohibit the *supply* of drugs for clinical trials which have not been authorised.

### Definition of a clinical trial

Having established the necessity to obtain a Clinical Trial Certificate it is important to clarify the activities which are included by this definition. In terms of the Medicines Act a clinical trial is 'an investigation consisting of the administration of a medicinal product by a doctor or dentist to patients where there is evidence that the product may have effects which are beneficial to the patient and the administration is for the purpose of determining whether, or to what extent, the product has that effect or any other, whether beneficial or harmful'. The definition stresses the potential benefit to the patient and for this reason investigations in healthy subjects to study the pharmacokinetics or pharmacodynamics of a new drug are specifically excluded since no benefit is expected. No notification or authorisation is necessary in these circumstances.

Healthy subjects are not automatically excluded since trials in such persons who may benefit come within the terms of the Act: For example, a Clinical Trial Certificate is necessary before a trial of an oral contraceptive or a trial of an influenza vaccine is conducted since in both situations a potential benefit exists.

This definition serves to make a reasonable distinction between those trials which require authorisation and those which do not. Certain difficulties may arise in some trials where no benefit to the patient may be expected (for example, in the investigation of a beta-blocking drug in asthmatics to determine its selectivity). It is suggested that in difficult cases the proposed studies should be discussed with the professional staff of Medicines Division. From a practical point of view, trials involving patients are generally subject to Clinical Trial Certificate requirements.

Occasionally some trials, such as consumer studies, may not be supervised by a doctor or dentist and in these circumstances it is necessary for the supplier to hold a Product Licence rather than a Clinical Trial Certificate.

### Application for a Clinical Trial Certificate

The Licensing Authority do not lay down rigid requirements concerning the data which must be provided before authorisation can be given for the clinical trial of a new drug. It issues guide-lines for applicants. This subject has already been adequately reviewed (Griffin 1974).

Essentially the application will consist of a detailed clinical trial protocol together with supporting experimental animal data. The latter will include: the chemistry, pharmacy and pharmacology which provide information on the quality of the new drug and its range of pharmacological activity; pharmacokinetic studies in animals which provide information on the likely absorption, distribution and excretion in man; preliminary metabolic studies in man which may also have been performed. Other data received at this stage will include acute and chronic toxicity studies and information on possible effects on reproduction. Taken together these data give information on the therapeutic potential of the new drug and on its likely margin of safety. Details of any clinical studies performed abroad are relevant and will also be submitted.

These data are assessed by the professional pharmaceutical and medical staff of Medicines Division, and is then referred to the relevant Sub-Committees of the

Committee on Safety of Medicines. Most applications are referred to the Sub-Committee on Chemistry, Pharmacy and Standards and to the Sub-Committee on Toxicity, Clinical Trials and Therapeutic Efficacy. A separate Sub-Committee on Biological Substances considers Clinical Trials Certificate applications for drugs which cannot be adequately characterised by chemical means, such as hormones, blood products and vaccines. If the data are considered to be satisfactory, the Committee on Safety of Medicines will advice that a Clinical Trial Certificate can be issued by the Licensing Authority for the supply of the drug for the specific trials and clinical indications detailed in the application. Extension of studies to other clinical centres or for other clinical indications will require separate authorisation; such matters can usually be dealt with expediently.

It is important to note that the holder of the certificate has an obligation to inform the Licensing Authority of any serious or unexpected adverse reactions which occur in the course of the trial.

## Special circumstances

It has previously been mentioned that there are certain circumstances in which a Clinical Trial Certificate is not necessary, namely for investigations in healthy subjects who are unlikely to benefit. In this section, other special circumstances are considered.

A Clinical Trial Certificate is not necessary if a doctor wishes to use a new but unauthorised drug on his own responsibility for the treatment of individual named patients. Secondly, no certificate is required for a clinical trial on a marketed product for a clinical indication authorised in the licence or where an individual clinician undertakes a trial on a marketed product without asking the manufacturer to make supplies specially available. This reflects the policy that it is not the trial which is controlled but the *supply* of the drug for the trial; this protects the freedom of the clinician to use any available drug for any purpose which he considers appropriate.

An alternative procedure applies when the trial is not to be conducted under arrangements made by the pharmaceutical company concerned and the clinician requests that a drug be made available which is not already available to him in the form required. Providing no objection is raised by the Licensing Authority, the supplier may be granted an exemption from the need to hold a Clinical Trial Certificate to make the drug available to the clinician. Under these regulations, the clinician signs a declaration that the trial is being conducted on his own initiative and has not been arranged by the pharmaceutical company. The most usual circumstances in which this exemption applies is for the supply of identical tablets or capsules of marketed products in order to carry out a double-blind trial. I must emphasise that this procedure is not normally applicable to new drugs.

## Summary

Under the Medicines Act (1968), authorisation in the form of a Clinical Trial Certificate is necessary before a drug can be supplied for clinical trial patients. No authorisation is required for studies in healthy subjects where no benefit is expected or for clinical trials of marketed drugs in the indications specified on the product licence. Since the Act essentially controls the supply of drugs, a doctor may use an available drug for any purpose he considers appropriate including a clinical trial. In addition, no authorisation is necessary for the supply of an unauthorised drug for the *treatment* of individual named patients.

REFERENCE

Griffin, J.P. (1974) Requirements to be fulfilled before instituting clinical trials on new drugs. *Proceedings of the Royal Society of Medicine,* **67**, 581 - 584.

# 3. Volunteer Studies and Human Pharmacology— Phase I

I. M. JAMES

The main aim of early volunteer studies should be to evaluate all pharmacological properties of the drug in man so as to maximise its therapeutic impact. Having said this, however, the objectives of volunteer studies must be seen in the general context of the complete development of the drug. The problems must not be considered in isolation. Observations made during this early phase will certainly influence the design of later phases and indeed should even provoke further animal experiments.

Before dealing with the design of early volunteer studies it is necessary to consider who the clinical investigators should ideally be and to determine where exactly these volunteer studies should be performed.

## Selection of investigators and site

The selection of investigators and of location are interlinked problems. The following facilities appear desirable and some of them are essential. To some extent they are dependant on the type of study being done and the stage which it has reached.

Instruments are necessary to collect the appropriate pharmacological data.

A sufficient number of trained assistants, physicians, technicians and nursing staff are necessary. They should be able not only to cope with routine collection of data but also able to deal with any emergency situation that might arise.

Special investigation rooms are desirable. A calm quiet environment is important. Hospital wards with their associated activity are not usually suitable for performing such studies. Some control over the room temperature is also important especially in pharmacodynamic studies.

The investigators should be able to observe the subjects for an adequate period of time. The study must not have to stop at 5 p.m.

There is always danger when a new compound is given for the first time to man. The investigator must therefore have the ability and equipment to combat any untoward reaction. In 1976 this means that at least the initial studies should be done in a hospital environment. In my opinion any other decision has allowed arguments of convenience or of finance to outweigh those of safety for the volunteer.

The clinical investigator has to be both pharmacologist and physician. Whether or not he chooses to call himself a clinical pharmacologist is immaterial. He must understand the details of the animal pharmacology and toxicology and be able to assess the level of confidence with which the prehuman pharmacological conclusions have been drawn. Otherwise he is not in a position to fully understand the risk to which he is subjecting his volunteers. 'Doctors with no pharmacological training or those who are not willing to collaborate with a pharmacologist and adhere strictly to a protocol', according to Dengler (1974), 'very often underestimate the responsibility they are taking and are often of a potential danger to the subject'.

The professional clinical pharmacologist in a specialised hospital unit is the ideal investigator since he can function as physician yet be able to understand all the pharmacological problems involved. From the results of his observations he may be able to suggest further animal experiments. Occasionally investigations are performed by a 'systems specialist'. The danger of this is that undue attention may be focussed on one system of the body to the detriment of the others. Important pharmacological points of therapeutic relevance may be missed. One is likely to find only what one looks for. If the individual has had training in clinical pharmacology, in addition to his specialist training, then these strictures do not apply. The contribution of a systems specialist is usually found more helpful at a later phase.

There are many excellent clinical investigators in industry who have limited or no access to hospital facilities. This state of affairs must be changed. Clinical pharma-cologists in the health service are few and far between. At present they are principally concentrated in academic units in teaching hospitals. The importance of clinical pharmacology and the need for further clinical pharmacologists (although recognised by the Royal College of Physicians and by the Universities) has not resulted in the expected expansion of the subject, mainly for economic reasons. If better facilities are to be provided then much of the funding will need to come from industry, at least for the next few years.

The relationship between industry and academic units must be further improved. Secondment of individuals from industry to academic units and from academic units to industry needs to be encouraged. Such measures are consistent with the opinion of the Joint Committee on Higher Medical Training.

### The selection of subjects

Volunteer subjects are usually recruited from industrial personnel or from labora-tory staff in academic units. Such sources may become exhausted fairly rapidly. There is a real need for volunteers from other sources. One answer would be to set up a national register of volunteers similar to the register of blood donors, as suggested by Paul Turner, Professor of Clinical Pharmacology at St. Bartholomew's Hospital Medical School.

The volunteer should not be in a position of subservience to the investigator. For this reason many medical schools do not allow their students to volunteer for studies in academic clinical pharmacology units. Surely these doctors are adult enough to make such decisions for themselves? They can avoid the problem by acting as volunteers at other schools. The question of payment is difficult. Certainly the subject should not be 'out of pocket' for being public spirited, but neither should payment be so generous that it results in the 'professional' volunteer. It must not be so large as to be considered in any way a bribe. Once the subject has volunteered it is important that he or she is given a thorough medical examination by an independent doctor and that the subject's liver and renal function is shown to be normal. It is wise to inform the general practitioner of the volunteer that the study is being done.

It is important also that everyone taking part in a Phase I study is covered by adequate insurance. This applies to both the subject and the investigator.

## Ethics

Written consent after full explanation of the procedure in the presence of a witness is almost essential. Recently it has been suggested that verbal consent before the third party who confirms it in writing might be a satisfactory alternative to written consent. Nearly all research departments have now to submit the details of the projected investigation to an independent ethics committee composed of both professional and lay members. One effective system is that the protocol is sent to every member of the committee. They then return this with either their individual approval or adverse comments to the secretary. Any query is directed immediately to the investigator who can usually satisfy the committee member on the point fairly quickly. A full committee meeting is called only if a point of disagreement arises. This system causes little delay to the research project yet the ethics are competently and fully dealt with.

## Design of investigation

The design of the initial human investigation will be largely but not entirely dependent on the potential use of the drug; for instance, whether it is going to be used in the cardiovascular, respiratory or psychiatric fields. Only generalizations about the design are therefore possible. Ideally, both pharmacokinetic and pharmacodynamic measurements will be made. Apparent pharmacodynamic failure can be due to pharmacokinetic factors. If a drug lacks effect it is essential to discover the reason, for it may simply have failed to reach the site of action (Laurence, 1972). One of the objectives of initials experiments is to determine whether the pharmacological findings in animals apply also to man. In addition, special attention should be paid to those variables where animal experimentation is unable to supply the answer, for instance psychological testing.

Some of the more important factors influencing the design of volunteer studies are listed below:

The likely mechanism of action of the drug. If this is known from the animal experiments it is important to check whether the same conclusions apply for man. If the mechanism of action is known one can predict more accurately where and when the drug will be of clinical value and possibly be able to predict and avoid adverse reactions. The design of the investigation also is very much simplified.

The predicted effect is likely to occur after a single dose or after repeated administration. In the latter case prolonged studies involving continuous administration may be necessary in Phase I or may be more appropriate in Phase II.

The predicted effect is likely to occur only in diseased subjects. This does not necessarily preclude volunteer studies. An example of where acute volunteer studies are of use is afforded by pharmacokinetic studies involving antimicrobial drugs. Checks can be made to ascertain whether or not an adequate drug concentration is achieved in plasma, urine or at other appropriate sites.

The effect to be measured is the therapeutic effect itself or whether it is only believed to correlate with it. These latter studies are never easy to design well and interpretation of results is often difficult. There are some situations where normal volunteers are not used, for instance with cytotoxic drugs.

## Drug administration

### Acute data

On empirical grounds it is usually regarded as satisfactory if the drug is administered for one to four weeks in animals before a single dose or series of doses on one occasion is given to man. It is usual to start with two per cent of the scaled dose that is effective in animals and to double this until either the therapeutic effect occurs or the expected dose is reached. The route must be the same in animals and man. It is important to note that a minute dose of the radioactively labelled drug may be all that is necessary for initial pharmacokinetic data. However, it is better to correlate pharmacodynamic with pharmacokinetic changes and this can only be done with an effective dose. If possible the dose of the drug should be titrated against the effect. Such studies give much more information than a single fixed dose study.

### Chronic data

Long term treatment in man must be preceded by three to twelve months of toxicity testing in animals. This animal toxicity testing is designed to show the clinical pharmacologist or toxicologist what organ systems to monitor rather than to provide a testimonial for the drug. Therefore, the clinical pharmacologist will want to ensure that an adequate dose has been given to the animals.

With a single dose the rate of absorption as well as the fraction of drug absorbed from the dosage form can markedly influence the onset, intensity and duration of the response. With continuous administration on the other hand, the rate of absorption would have little effect on the plasma concentration and pharmacological effect achieved: In this case the major determinant of the steady state level would be the fraction of drug absorbed from the dosage form (Azarnoff 1972). The route or routes chosen for the study should be the ones by which it is intended that the drug should be given clinically. Variation in the route can result in surprising pharmacokinetic pharmacodynamic differences.

## Measurements

The measurements that will be made depend largely on the drug and the disease for which it was developed. It is important to set the net wide to check whether the same features are found in man as in animals and to evaluate whether there are any new ones which did not show up in the animal experiment. Particularly important is the testing of variables which are difficult or impossible to do in animals, for instance psychological testing. Good simple measurements that are unlikely to go wrong are more useful than complicated ones which are often found to be unreliable. For example, intelligent use of blood pressure measurements, pulse rates before and after exercise can reveal a lot more information than single readings or complicated measurements of cardiac function. Electrocardiography, electroencephalography and the use of radioisotopes including the inert radioactive gases can however provide a great deal of information with relatively little trauma. Safety lies in good experimental design using techniques with which the investigators are happy. An attempt should be made to correlate pharmacodynamic data with pharmacokinetic data.

In acute studies, estimation of plasma concentration provides clues as to whether the drug or a metabolite is responsible for the pharmacological effect, and will reveal whether the drug disappearance obeys first or zero order kinetics. The volume of distribution and clearance will be obtained for most drugs. Possibly the dosage schedule can be decided at this stage. The chronic administration pharmacokinetic data will serve as a check on initial impressions from the acute data and will allow more complicated pharmacokinetic systems to be revealed. If the kinetic data correlate well with the dynamic data there is strong presumptive evidence that the drug itself and not a breakdown product is responsible for the effect. If a more active metabolite is identified, the possibility of developing that compound as the drug of choice should be considered.

During chronic administration to volunteers monitoring of the function of those organs most likely to be affected (according to the animal data) should be performed. If a serious reaction occurs, such as jaundice, which may or may not be due to the drug it is essential to investigate the patient and circumstances as thoroughly as possible. Future subjects may be put at hazard unnecessarily or a useful drug may be withdrawn unnecessarily for want of evidence which would have been available if the adverse reaction had been properly investigated at the time (Dollery and Davies, 1970).

Although not often carried out during Phase I, the problems of possible drug interaction can frequently be answered by good human investigation. It is also important to know whether the drug acts as an enzyme inducer before it is given to patients on any large scale.

Complete records of all patients receiving the new drug must be kept. It is a good idea to design and print a proforma so that no details are forgotten for an individual. Time spent on the design of such forms will be amply rewarded during the stage of data analysis. Such information should be made available to workers investigating the drug in other centres.

I would like to repeat the plea of Modell (1974) that the results of Phase I studies be made available to everyone more quickly and especially when for some reason the drug is withdrawn. Knowledge will be more quickly disseminated and advances in the field of clinical pharmacology hastened.

## Conclusions

The main aim of early volunteer studies should be to evaluate all the pharmacological properties of the drug in man so as to maximise its therapeutic impact. In practice simple pharmacokinetic data such as half life and the volume of distribution should be obtained initially, in addition to the principal pharmacodynamic effects. More sophisticated investigations should be left to a later stage. Fuller collaboration of clinical pharmacologists in academic units, the health service, and the pharmaceutical industry will improve the speed, efficiency and safety with which such studies can be done.

REFERENCES

Azarnoff, D.L. (1972) Pharmacokinetics and bioavailability. In *Clinical Pharmacological Evaluation in Drug Control.* Heidelberg Symposium pp41 - 42. W.H.O. Regional Office for Europe and Copenhagen.

Dengler, H.J. (1972) Early human trials. Selection of investigators and subjects. Ibid. pp. 29 - 36.

Dollery, C.T. and Davies, D.S. (1970) Conduct of initial drug studies in man. *British Medical Bulletin,* December 1970 pp 232 - 236.

Laurence, D.R. (1972) Pharmacodynamic and pharmacokinetic information needed in early human drug studies. *Clinical Pharmacological Evaluation in Drug Control.* Heidelberg Symposium pp 37 - 40. W.H.O. Regional Office for Europe and Copenhagen.

Modell, W. (1974) Failed and Flawed Drugs: A Frozen Resource. Ch. I. In *Principles and Techniques of Human Research and Therapeutics.* Ed. F. Gilbert McMahon Ch. 1, pp 1 - 3, Futura Publications.

# 4. Clinical Trials— Phases II, III and IV

R. B. SMITH

Although this chapter is entitled 'Clinical Trials - Phases II, III and IV' it is important to consider more than the purely mechanical activities associated with clinical trials. The following is intended to be a guide, necessarily superficial, to some of the objectives and processes of clinical research together with the philosophy behind these. At the outset two important points must be continually borne in mind. Firstly, clinical research on a potential new medicine must constitute a continuous co-ordinated programme of study. This will extend beyond the actual marketing of the substance and must last for as long as it is used by man. Secondly, such a programme must be truly international to enable maximum benefit to be derived.

In this chapter the clinical trials programme is examined under three headings: Why? What? and How? Particular emphasis is placed on the first two of these questions since if the reasons for monitoring the trials and the questions being asked of the drug are clearly delineated at the outset this will point to the critical feature of trial design.

## Why?

If a man will begin with certainties he shall end in doubts, but if he will be content to begin with doubts he shall end in certainties.

F. Bacon     1561 - 1626

The paramount reason for initiating clinical research is to confirm in man the useful properties of new drugs which may be predicated by preclinical tests. In other words the objective is to produce new knowledge. As Fisher (1936) wrote: 'New knowledge comes from experience by inductive inference and is the only way from which it can come'. By creating this new knowledge we hope to identify possible benefits and possible dangers to human beings which may arise either directly or indirectly from the use of the new medicine. Although it has often been correctly observed that the treatment of every patient is virtually an experiment, it is none the less true that the greater the previous experience the less is the chance of a totally unexpected result.

Every patient experience with a new medicine is essentially a clinical trial but the term has been defined by an ABPI working party (1974) more broadly as:

'A clinical trial is a scientific experiment in which a drug or procedure is applied with diagnostic, therapeutic or prophylactic intent to patients. It is part of clinical pharmacology but stresses the clinical benefit'.

To make this definition even more complete we should add the word 'device' as many current developments fall within this category. In initiating a clinical research programme consisting of clinical trials of varying complexity we are attempting to quantify the degree of safety and efficacy of the new substance. Any therapeutically active substance is bound to have some degree of risk associated with it by virtue of its activity which implies that it is capable of modifying body processes. The aim in clinical research is to progress from a state of virtually no knowledge to complete knowledge. Complete knowledge is only attainable, if at all, after a considerable period of time.

This progression is represented in Figure 4.1.

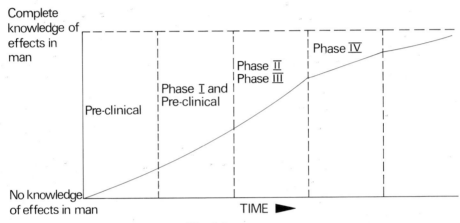

Fig. 4.1

The time course of clinical development prior to marketing will depend to a great extent on what is being investigated but phase IV will last for as long as the subject is used by man.

The decision to try a new drug in man will be based upon animal and human pharmacology and animal toxicity data. However, Litchfield (1962) has surveyed the value of animal screens in predicting toxicity and found that of 89 different drug effects monitored, 33 were seen *only* in man. He concluded that there was no basis for predicting these effects from animals.

The decision to proceed to man is finely balanced since toxicity in animals may not be reproduced in man and conversely the absence of toxicity in animals does not indicate a no-risk situation in humans. Only carefully monitored *human* experience can give a fully valid view of the risk : benefit ratio. The question of safety and toxicity in relation to efficacy is complex since none of these parameters is absolute. This is illustrated in Figure 4.2.

Drug A may be considered a safe and very effective medicine, the ideal drug. It is the profile for which to aim in selecting drugs intended to be taken by man for many years. Example B on the other hand is less safe than A and less effective. It may be useful for a narrow range of diseases or in patients who cannot tolerate drug A. Drug C comes within the same category as B but with greater toxicity. D on the

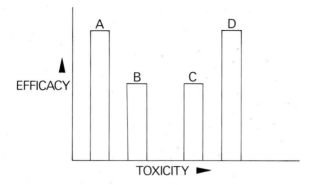

## SAFETY/TOXICITY in relation to EFFICACY

A = safe and very effective
B = more toxicity and less effectiveness
C = appreciable toxicity same efficacy as B
D = significant toxicity but as effective as A

Fig 4.2

other hand is very effective but very toxic. Risk versus benefit has to be carefully considered and drug D might be, for instance, very active as an anti-cancer agent. Consequently the risks may be justifiable. Exact quantification of such properties relative to risk would be the object of a clinical research programme with these as with any other new drug.

## What?

At the 18th World Medical Assembly (1964), under the general heading of 'clinical research combined with professional care' it was resolved that in the treatment of the sick person, the doctor must be free to use a new therapeutic measure if, in his judgement, it offers hope of saving life, re-establishing health or alleviating suffering. This definition is as relevant when applied to medical advisers in the pharmaceutical industry as it is to the practising physician. It gives the justification for the search for new knowledge that Fisher alluded to.

A co-ordinated clinical research programme will develop in relation to a new drug:

Indications for use
Dosage range in relation to indications
Presence or absence of side actions which may be: harmful
                                                beneficial
Presence or absence of drug interactions which may consist of: antagonism
                                                              additive effects
                                                              synergistic effects
Pharmacokinetics in different populations

Paediatric applications bearing in mind that children are not merely 'small adults'.

A few years ago clinical trials were designated:

Initial

Confirmatory

Marketing or commercial.

It was, and still is in some spheres, usual to regard the former two as 'clinical research' with its respectable overtones while the latter was regarded as 'medical service' with a slightly less reputable connotation. Such a definition is wholly false. It may be convenient to divide personnel supervising pre-marketing studies from those concerned with post-marketing studies but the objectives of both groups are precisely the same in terms of striving to acquire complete knowledge of the new drug.

Clinical trials activity is now generally considered under four phases. Phase I has been discussed in the previous chapter. The essential difference between phase I and later phases is that phase I uses healthy volunteers whereas phases II, III and IV use patients with varying degrees of illness. Although there are differing legal views on the validity of informed consent both healthy individuals and patients must volunteer for the studies within the terms of the Declaration of Helsinki (1964).

### Phase II studies

The primary purpose of these trials is to examine whether a new drug is effective for one (or more) clinical indications. These studies commence when patients rather than healthy subjects are used for the first time.

These early investigations may be uncontrolled. In the past such studies have been decried, but properly conducted they can contribute much valuable information. More will be said about this later. The studies must be adequate to permit an early estimate of the risk benefit ratio. They can furnish information on unwanted effects together with an estimation of clinical efficacy in relation to drug concentrations in body fluids and tissues (pharmacokinetics). Elimination of the drug from the body (performed also in phase I investigations) should be checked also in patients as they may handle the drug differently due to modified bodily function (pharmacodynamics).

Careful study even at this early stage may show a novel indication. Such a finding can occur at any stage of the clinical programme (including late phase IV) and the possibility must be constantly borne in mind when the total experience with the agent is being sifted.

Early studies are the safest since they start with single small doses of the new drug in only a few patients who are closely monitored. Progression to multiple dose phase II studies with expansion of the patient population is built upon early reassuring experience with the new drug.

### Phase III studies

The decision to proceed to Phase III investigations is taken when the clinical researcher is convinced that an acceptable risk profile in relation to efficacy exists.

Therefore extended usage of the new drug can be justified with somewhat less supervision in a large number of patients. The progression is a gradual extension since supervision in early phase III studies is as close as that exercised in phase II. As confidence is increased and more patients become involved, supervision must necessarily be lessened. However it should never be at such a low level that patients are exposed to unnecessary hazards. The actual degree of supervision required will vary not only with the degree to which the programme has advanced but also with the particular drug being tested. As phase III progresses, many different types of trial design can be used. This will be referred to below.

The end result of a clinical trials programme must be to enable practising physicians to use the new drug competently and to its maximum advantage. To do this they must be able accurately to weigh the benefits against the risks in a variety of different cases. The indications and dosage must be confirmed and evidence must be available at the end of phase III studies which testifies to safety in chronic use where this is indicated. In order to answer the questions: Does the drug accumulate in the body? Does toxicity develop with extended usage? the incidence and severity of adverse reactions must be closely monitored. This is referred to in a later chapter.

*Phase IV studies*

The term phase IV is common usage but does not appear to have been adequately defined. A working definition is that it encompasses all those studies undertaken after obtaining a marketing licence.

Pre-marketing studies by their very nature leave important questions unanswered. For example the toxicity of any agent could not have been accurately assessed in clinical trial if the incidence of agranulocytosis was 1 in 20,000 or less. Yet it is important to know if it does occur. Phase II and III studies suffer from three major drawbacks:
Limited patient numbers
Limited duration of patient exposure
Restricted patient populations
Therefore phase IV studies should be designed to reveal:
Adverse reactions relative to chronic usage
Drug efficacy in long term use where, for instance, the course of a disease may be modified over a period of months or years
Additional comparative data of a long term nature
Non-responders. These can be examined in detail
New uses and indications
An assessment of overuse or misuse liability
An assessment of abuse liability
Drug interactions and compatibility with other agents since:
1. Metabolism may be increased
2. Metabolism may be decreased
3. Changes in urinary pH may affect the drug's excretion
4. There may be active tubular secretion
5. There may be inhibition of gut absorption

6. Alteration of gut motility may occur

7. Pharmacological interference, at for instance, nerve endings may result.

Thus phase IV studies have a number of reasons for existing unrelated to commercial motivation, although as the studies proceed much useful spin-off will occur.

*Clinical trial design*

So far only the broad objectives have been examined but now we must consider what methods to use in order to produce a meaningful result. All trial work must be effectively planned since it is pointless to expect badly formed questions and poorly planned experiments to give reliable answers.

*Uncontrolled trials.* Trials may be controlled or uncontrolled. In recent years controlled studies have achieved such a scientific reputation that many have thought that uncontrolled trials are either unreliable or even valueless. This is not true. Much useful information can be gained by well planned and conducted uncontrolled studies. They may answer more limited questions than do controlled studies but are just as important. When a new drug has been granted a marketing licence it will be used by the medical profession on an uncontrolled basis. It is therefore useful to be able to gauge its likely behaviour well before this event. In conditions having one hundred per cent mortality the reason for dispensing with an overt control is obvious. The term 'overt control' means that a degree of control has been exercised, in this instance historically. Such an early uncontrolled study is usually extremely stringent in that a new drug is tried first in all those patients who are either not responding or poorly responding to existing medications. By this process a degree of control has been introduced. Uncontrolled and controlled trials should not be considered as competitive but as complementary to each other.

Early phase II studies may be conducted as uncontrolled open (that is both patients and doctor are aware they are using a new medicine) trials and are designed to answer such questions as: Does it work? What is the most usual dose at which effects are observed and what adverse reactions, if any, are associated with this dosage? Basically uncontrolled studies will give an early view of the *technique* of therapy.

*Controlled trials.* The aim is to introduce a method of comparison between the new drug and an appropriate baseline which is usually either no treatment at all, a placebo or an appropriate treatment. The time course when this comparison is made must be either identical or compensated for to increase the validity of the results. It is for this reason that historical control is considered as an adjunct to uncontrolled rather than controlled studies. Control may also be exercised by influencing the types of patient admitted to trial. There are four main controlled trial designs:

1. *Matched pairs.* An attempt is made to standardize the patients by matching for as many of a series of physical and social characteristics (sex, age, size, race and class) as possible. Alternatively only patients with a particular type, severity or duration of illness may be selected. The course and progression of such illness is also important. This trial design is based on the assumption that pair matching of patients allows a more accurate comparison. There are many imperfections since no two patients are really alike. There are difficulties in accurately matching the pairs which may impair

patient recruitment and it may not be possible to treat each half of the pair at the same time. With conditions like angina this could be of critical importance.

2. *Cross-over design.* This employs the principle of the patient as his own control. A group of patients is selected and given both regimens for a set period of time. There are difficulties with carry-over effects from either treatment. The method cannot be used when one of the drugs is curative or the disease either is self limiting or alters radically within the trial period. Many of the problems can be minimised by randomising both the order of treatment and the entry of patients into the study, for example:

|  | Treatment Periods | | |
|---|:---:|:---:|:---:|
|  | 1 | 2 | 3 |
| Patient 1 | A | B | C |
| Patient 2 | B | C | A |
| Patient 3 | C | A | B |

This is a 3 x 3 latin square. It can be repeated so that at the end of the study equal numbers of patients should have had comparable treatment orders. This enables a valid comparison between the three treatments to be made.

3. *Group comparisons.* Patients are randomly allocated to groups and the groups are then assigned to a particular treatment. A possible drawback is that the groups may be wrongly selected. Proper selection depends on strict randomised entry into the trial. There are two major types of design for these studies, simple and factorial. The latter gives the more efficient use of a restricted patient population.

4. *Mixed designs.* Features of all the major trial designs can be incorporated. For instance, matched pairs can be selected, treated with one medication and then crossed over. Criteria and rules applied to patient selection can be augmented by controlling treatments. Historical or retrospective control has been discussed. There are three other methods available:

No treatment. Certain conditions are not suitable for ethical reasons.

Placebos. A pharmacologically inactive substance is given to patients to assess their response to the fact that they believe it has activity. Placebos can show peak effects, carry-over effects, cumulative effects and sometimes habituation and addiction. They may also show varying efficacy and the response may be either positive or negative. They can exhibit all the attributes of an active preparation for such is the power of suggestion. For this reason it may be worthwhile performing a pilot study in order to screen out placebo reactors.

Active drug. If this is modified for a double blind trial, steps must be taken to ensure that the modified active drug has comparable bioavailability and other properties to that which it would have under normal conditions of use.

If both doctor and patients are aware they are using a new drug the trial is open. In a single blind trial the patient will not know which treatment is which and in a double blind study neither the patient nor the physician knows. The latter bias is an attempt to neutralize bias in the trial arising from either the doctor's attitude to the patient or the patient's attitude to the doctor and the medication given. All treatments should be randomly allocated according to a pre-set code which is not broken except in an emergency.

How exactly treatments are matched depends on the drug being tested. If the new drug is formulated as a white tablet then placebos can be made to match. Where another active treatment is to be used for comparison, care must be exercised to ensure the matched formulation performs comparably in terms of bioavailability with the formulation used in medical practice. If, on the other hand, it is desired to compare dissimilar treatments, for example a tablet and an injection, then both placebo tablets and placebo injections would have to be employed. This is known as a double placebo (dummy) technique. It can be used to compare dissimilar preparations thereby avoiding the bioavailability problems mentioned.

In the past the concept of active placebos has been employed. These are really positive controls albeit often in homeopathic quantities.

Any clinical research programme seeks for a definite therapeutic response. The pilot study will have identified placebo responders so that they can be eliminated. The quantification of relative therapeutic efficacy can be difficult due to the unpre- dictability of human ailments. A negative result from a controlled clinical trial may not mean lack of clinical efficacy but that the patient population was inadequate, badly selected or the trial mismanaged. The objective must be to disprove the null hypothesis which states that the detection of a difference was a chance event and no real difference exists. It must be conslusively shown that the detection of a difference between treatments was *not* due to an accident of measurement or observation.

## How?

The first step is to frame precisely the questions it is proposed to answer. This is the first step in the preparation of a protocol. The questions should be written out in full. Next will come a statement of which type of study is considered to be most appropriate. Thirdly is the critical area of patient selection. Which patients are to be included must be defined, for instance type of disease, duration of disease, sex and age range. Patients to be specifically excluded are:

Patients of childbearing potential and those already pregnant

Minors unless this is specific to the trial

Those with a history of allergy

Those whose laboratory results fall outside the normal range.

A major stumbling block is failure to consider the number of patients who should be included in the trial to suit the design chosen. The wisest course is to consult a statistician before the trial so that correct numbers likely to give a positive answer are chosen, and the chances of a false negative due to inadequate numbers is reduced. If a sequential design is used this matters less since the trial runs until a definite trend appears as to which is the preferred treatment. In general, more trials suffer from too few patients than too many. Clark and Downie (1966) published graphs to help in the choice of numbers (Figs. 4.3 and 4.4).

Next the method of assessment to be used in the trial must be stated. This will include routine recording of biochemical and other bodily functions and a record of response to therapy. This may be objective or subjective or a mixture of both.

## NUMBER OF PATIENTS REQUIRED FOR CLINICAL TRIALS

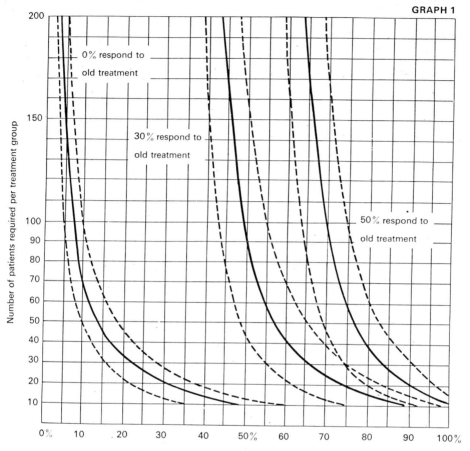

Fig. 4.3

Assessment may be on an open basis (even though the physician may not know which treatment is used) or blind by an observer who is not concerned in clinical supervision of the patients in the trial. Assessment of X-rays and ECGs lends itself to this approach.

Side effects should be monitored in every trial but there are different methods. There is a difference between side effects specifically asked for and those which are volunteered. Both should be followed. Side effects may be either desirable or undesirable and pleasant or unpleasant. It should not be forgotten that today's side effect may be the major indication for tomorrow's drug.

The success or failure of a trial or trial programme may depend on the degree and accuracy of recording data. This cannot be too greatly stressed. A practical balance must be struck between what degree of detail is ideal and what is practicable. This will depend on the questions which were originally asked in the protocol. It often helps if doctors are not involved in the filling in of records. People trained as clerks

NUMBER OF PATIENTS REQUIRED FOR CLINICAL TRIALS

50% CHANCE OF SUCCESS   5% LEVEL OF SIGNIFICANCE

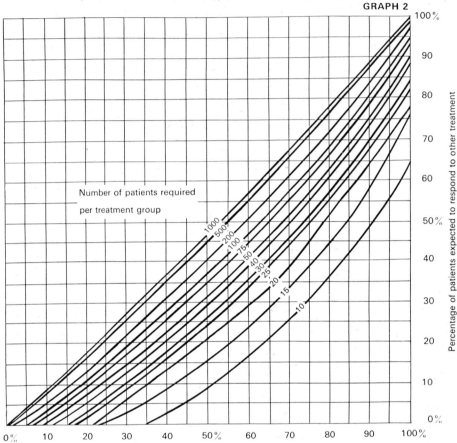

GRAPH 2

Number of patients required

per treatment group

Percentage of patients expected to respond to other treatment

Percentage of patients expected to respond to one treatment

Fig. 4.4

are usually much more conscientious and accurate. Simple check lists with such details as 'are the records properly identified for each patient and hospital?' are available in the literature.

The protocol must also contain details on the randomization, labelling and dosage of treatments and dispensing instructions. A superbly constructed and executed trial will still fail if the patients do not take the drugs. It is worthwhile building in checks to verify that the drugs are being taken properly. This can be done by spot blood checks, spot urine checks and tablet counting.

The question of writing up clinical research work is important. Whether a trial is eventually published or not, a written report should be made if only as a record for the company.

Finally Figure 4.5 gives a check list of some of the common causes of failure of clinical trials.

| Plan | Protocol | - wrong questions asked<br>- incorrect trial design |
|---|---|---|
| **Planners** | Statistician<br>Consultant<br>Medical adviser | - not consulted<br>- inexperienced, too busy<br>- inexperienced |
| **Powers** | Ethical committee<br>Consultant<br>Registrar | - delay<br>- loses interest<br>- over worked |
| **Pilots** | Medical adviser<br>Clinical trials team<br>Nurse observer | - inadequate follow-up<br>- badly managed<br>- badly motivated |
| **Passenger** | The therapeutic<br>substance | - badly formulated<br>- appearance of toxicity<br>- inadequate clinical trials stock |
| **Patients** | | - bad selection<br>- inadequate recruitment (Lasagna's Law)<br>- uncooperative, not taking medicines properly<br>- not attending for assessments |
| **Patients' records** | | - badly designed<br>- incompletely filled-in<br>- not properly identified |
| **Pharmacists** | Company<br><br>Hospitals | - faults in supply of clinical trial materials<br>- faults in dispensing of clinical trial materials |
| **Publishing** | | - lack of impetus to write up trial and submit to journal<br>- incomplete results<br>- poor writing up<br>- lack of journal space |

Fig. 4.5 Clinical trials. Some causes of delay and failure to complete.

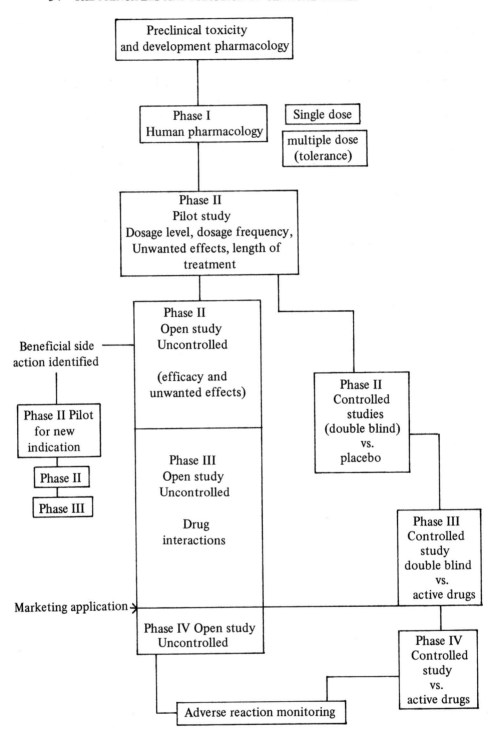

Fig. 4.6 Drug development

## Conclusion

The subject of clinical trials in phase II, III and IV is large and has only been briefly outlined here. I have included Figure 4.6 to show progression from uncontrolled studies to controlled studies versus placebo, and finally to controlled studies versus active drugs. How many patients need to be studied at each stage will depend on the particular drug being investigated. I have shown the uncontrolled open study continuing past the marketing stage so that a mechanism exists for further monitoring of the new drug. Thus data from patients who have been taking the agent continuously for several years would be available. The clinical research programme is not merely a mechanism to achieve registration of a new drug, it is a process of governing new knowledge which is critical to the safety of man and the guidance of the medical profession. To achieve this it must be continuously in existence on an international basis.

## REFERENCES

Medicopharmaceutical Forum (1974) A report by the Forum's working party on clinical trials. London : Medicopharmaceutical Forum. p.7.

Clark, C.J. & Downie, C.C. (1966) A method for the rapid determination of the number of patients to include in a controlled clinical trial. *Lancet,* **ii**, 1357.

Litchfield, J.T. (1962) Symposium on clinical drug evaluation and human pharmacology. XVI : Evaluation of the safety of new drugs by means of tests in animals. *Clinical Pharmacology and Therapeutics,* **3**, 665.

World Medical Association (1964) Declaration of Helsinki. *British Medical Journal,* **i**, 177.

Fisher, R.A. (1936) Statistical Methods for Research Workers. 6th Ed. London : Oliver & Boyd.

## FURTHER READING

Amery, W. & Dony, J. (1975) A clinical trial design avoiding undue placebo treatment. *Journal of Clinical Pharmacology,* **15**, 674.

Bradford Hill, Sir A.(1971) *Principles of Medical Statistics.* 9th Ed. London: Lancet.

Goldenthal, E.I. (1968) Current views on safety evaluation of drugs. *F.D.A. Papers.*

Green, F.K.H. (1954) The clinical evaluation of remedies. *Lancet,* **ii**, 1085.

Hamilton, M. (1961) *Lectures on the Methodology of Clinical Research.* London: Livingstone.

Harris, E.L. & Fitzgerald, J.D. (Eds.) (1970) *The Principles and Practice of Clinical Trials.* London: Livingstone.

Jouhar, A.J. & Grayson, M.F. (Eds.) (1973) *International Aspects of Drug Evaluation and Usage.* London: Churchill Livingstone.

Lear, J.A., Rudolfo, A.S., Decker, J.L. & Paulus, H. (1970) *Anti:inflammatory (Non-Steroidal Drugs).* Pharmaceutical Manufacturer's Association.

Marsh, B.T. (1974) Clinical trials procedures - a summary of requirements in 33 countries. *Journal of International Medical Research,* **2**, 26.

Maxwell, Cyril (1973) *Clinical Research for All.* Cambridge Medical Publications.

National Academy of Sciences (1975) Report of workshop on clinical trials of drugs. *Clinical Pharmacology and Therapeutics,* **18** (5) Part 2.

Soleri, M.F. & Wheatley, D. (1966) A method of combining the results of several clinical trials. *Clinical Trials Journal,* **3**, 537.

Symposium (1966) Measurement in therapeutic assessment. *Proceedings of the Royal Society of Medicine,* **59**, Suppl.

Tabor, B-Z. (1969) *Proving New Drugs: a Guide to Clinical Trials* Los Altos, California.

Wardell, M. & Lasagna, L. (1975) Regulation and drug development. *Evaluative Studies,* American Enterprise Institute.

Zaimis, Eleanor (Ed.) (1963) *Evaluation of New Drugs in Man.* Oxford: Pergamon.

# Discussion Part I

*Dr. D.M. Burley (CIBA):* I would like to ask Professor Vere about the possible waste of human resource in carrying out trials of 'me too' drugs in large numbers. If we only had one beta blocker our knowledge would be limited. How many should we have? Would you accept one or two, five or six? Is thirty too many?

*Professor Vere:* Perhaps you should refer to Chapter 1 where I said that there is a transition point in ethical considerations. This point is where the sheer momentum of drug development takes over as the primary driving force. This can be dangerous. We should keep to the prime objective which is the development of compounds of new theoretical or practical interest.

*Dr. P.J. Roylance (M.S. & D.):* The ethical aims of a new drug should be either a novel mode of action or superior activity. A compound which is exactly the same as others but with improved safety should be worth putting on the market.

I would contest that trials in children should wait until after trials in adults. Children are not just small adults but different human beings.

*Professor Vere:* Your first point is discussed more fully in Chapter 1. Superiority includes safety, efficacy and palatability.

With regard to trials in children, I agreed that it would be better if we could do some trials in children, but sometimes this is not possible. An obvious example is that you can not treat cancer in people without cancer whether they are children or adults.

*Chairman:* A few years ago the College produced a report on studies in volunteers. It was felt that research ought to include children and mentally handicapped people. There was trouble with the Department of Health. A letter was sent to all practitioners saying that, according to legal advice, it was illegal to do any research with children or mentally handicapped people. No one could give permission for such studies. At a meeting a year ago, a lawyer spoke to chairmen from all ethical committees about the legal position. He said that it had never been tested in the courts, and that nothing would ever come from a Court action.

*Professor Vere:* Sir Harvey Druitt's rules are illustrated in the following diagram:

## RESEARCH IN CHILDREN

Parents may not consent if there is an experiment of 'no particular benefit *and* which may cause some risk of harm'.

*(Sir Harvey Druitt's ruling).*

The parent cannot consent if there is no individual benefit and if there is a risk or danger. The parent has to understand this and so does the Regulatory Body. Parental consent need not be sought if there is no risk or if individual benefit is to be expected. The problems are that most parents do not or cannot understand the rules, and that no-one can predict or evaluate discomfort or danger on a trial.

*Chairman:* Should ethical committees follow up research and assess the progress of trials?

*Professor Vere:* Ethical committees tend to isolate themselves from the investigators. I would like to see ethical committees follow through a trial to assess the outcome. If they do not do this, how else can they correct their procedures. They should be the investigator's friend and critic.

*Mr. J.J. Grimshaw (Aldershot):* The collection of widespread information from general practitioners once a drug has been marketed is a predominantly marketing exercise. It is not a scientific exercise but how else is a company going to get back information on the wide use of the drug? There is otherwise no definite feed back of this sort of information.

*Professor Vere:* I would agree. I was one of a group of people who suggested a monitored release of drugs. What is wrong is that there is no preliminary stage between trials of a drug and its general release for marketing. But what would happen if every company did widespread clinical surveys? At present there is no gap between Phase 3 and Phase 4 studies. The patent law may have to be reviewed. It may have to be changed to give sliding patents with protection during a vulnerable pre-marketing phase of drug use so that a company would not be penalised. The present patent laws tie us down.

*Dr. D.M. Burley (CIBA):* Dr. Cuthbert, it is sometimes difficult to differentiate between a healthy volunteer and a sick patient. When a woman with postmenopause symptoms is given oestrogen, we are treating a physiological process. Is she a volunteer or a patient?

*Dr. Cuthbert:* If a drug is administered for a medicinal purpose and we expect a therapeutic response, even if it is a prophylactic one, then we must assume that we are dealing with a patient.

*Dr. P.J. Roylance ( M.S. & D.):* The Food and Drug Administration (USA) define a normal human volunteer as one who is not receiving any treatment at all.

*Professor Vere:* The FDA definition is not always the rule in this country. If someone is complaining of a symptom, then they should be regarded as a patient. For example, a patient with exercise induced asthma when without symptoms is still a patient.

*Dr. R.K. Rondel (Bristol Myers):* Dr. Cuthbert, if one gives asthmatic subjects beta blockers to evaluate the effects on the bronchi, would one need a clinical trial certificate (CTC)?

*Dr. Cuthbert:* A clinical trial is an investigation where benefit is expected. If a trial might result in any harm, then it might require a CTC.

*Dr. B. Boeree (M.S. & D.):*  Following your observation that potential benefit to the patient should be mandatory for admission to a clinical trial, would you comment on the situation where parallel groups are studied and the patients in one group receive placebo only?

*Dr. Cuthbert:*  It is generally accepted that the placebo group is an important part of the clinical trial. This group must be seen in the context of the whole trial.

*Dr. C.C. Downie (ICI):*  Dr. Cuthbert, can you undertake a clinical trial without a CTC if all patients are named?

*Dr. Cuthbert:*  No. Named patients are excluded from the Medicines Act because it is realised that doctors may wish to treat individual patients from specific therapeutic purposes. Doctors who request drugs from companies for therapeutic purposes need not necessarily be conducting clinical trials. If you supply material for a number of named patients, this could be published and look like a clinical trial.

*Chairman:*  Thalidomide is very effective in lepromatous leprosy and is now almost impossible to obtain. Was there a clinical trial to find this effect?

*Dr. Cuthbert:*  There was no clinical trial but it is well known in the Hospital of Tropical Medicine that it is effective and available for this particular purpose.

*Dr. A.M. Edwards (Fisons):*  You said that you are hoping for a turn round of four to five months for CTC applications. Will there be a guarantee of five to six months and no longer?

*Dr. Cuthbert:*  Assuming the application is alright, then yes. Delays occur because questions have to be asked. Companies are approached for additional information. If applications are straight forward, then there should be no delay.

*Dr. W.L. Burland (Smith Kline & French):*  One aspect which Dr. James did not cover was the protection that one might offer volunteers. If a general register of volunteers is formed, one will have to provide insurance cover for volunteers against the unforeseen occurrence.

*Dr. James:*  I think that adequate insurance of the volunteer is very important. I would repeat that, if we are able to get a national register, insurance along these lines or by this sort of body may be possible.

*Chairman:*  A word about undergraduate volunteers. This is a common problem in Liverpool because some medical practitioners have used medical undergraduate volunteers. I think this is undesirable for the reasons that Dr. James has said; but on the other hand undergraduates are convenient volunteers. We have ruled that undergraduate volunteers should come from different faculties, so that they are not subjected to the stresses or rewards that Dr. James has mentioned.

*Dr. James:*  I agree with you. I would also point out the educational aspect. I remember taking part in an early volunteer study when I was a medical student.

I learnt much about thyroid function tests during this time. I kept asking the investigator what was happening, how all the tests were done and how various things were developed. I think that there is a variable educative role which we should not forget. Your arguments would probably be more relevant to the medical student 10 or 15 years ago. I think that today's medical students perhaps have not quite the same verve.

*Dr. W. Bogie (Hoechst):* I was interested in the way that your ethical committee is run so that they may send out a protocol without having a full committee meeting. We have lay members on our ethical committee. I would think it very difficult for them to judge adequately a protocol that was sent round. I feel that the lay members of an ethical committee act like a patient's friend. They need full explanation of a protocol probably in the committee situation. Therefore although you find your system helpful, I would say that it is not the best one for us.

*Dr. James:* There are easy ways round that. The lay members have someone to interpret the data for them. The data is sent out and then interpreted. This is what we do. If they want to discuss the protocol with the investigator, then they are encouraged to do so. Sometimes it is simpler to show such a person the apparatus that one is using rather than to give an explanation in a committee room.

*Dr. R.A.P. Burt (Lilly Research):* Dr. James, you said 'if there are no blood levels then it is hardly surprising that the drug does not work'. This has an appealing simplicity but it is dangerous to dogmatise. For example, nalorphine and cyclazine produce their central nervous system effects long after the drug has apparently disappeared from the blood. A drug that is used to treat urinary tract infection might be concentrated in the urine long after it has left the blood. A drug may produce its action solely through its metabolites: There may be no parent substance in the blood but activity may still be present.

You partly answered this by pointing out the importance of really understanding what the trial is for. I feel the same degree of planning should go into human pharmacological studies. The reasons for doing blood level studies should be clearly understood so that at the end of the study we know the value of the blood level data.

*Dr. James:* Yes, nearly, but fortunately the event did not occur. We gave isoprenaline really talking in general terms. I might have made too great a generalisation.

*Dr. C.C. Downie (I.C.I.):* We have a clinical pharmacology unit within our research department and our volunteers come from the staff. I think we meet all the criteria that you have mentioned, perhaps in some respects even more in that the volunteers may actually see the animal experiments. But we cannot meet your last criterion. Ours are not hospital premises and you strongly stressed that these experiments should be carried out in hospitals. In your own experience have any events occurred in hospital which would have been dangerous if you had not been on hospital premises?

*Dr. James:* Yest, nearly, but fortunately the even did not occur, We gave isoprenaline to someone who had had an untoward reaction to it, having alerted the services, but fortunately nothing happened. I think this is a difficult problem. I have great sympathy with your situation. But again I must emphasis that in my opinion the very earliest studies should be done in hospital, in case something goes wrong.

*Dr. C.F. Speirs (Lilly Research):* Would Dr. James advise us how often in one year a volunteer should be allowed to take part in a human pharmacological study?

*Dr. James:* I must beg the question because it depends on exactly what one is doing. If it is a fairly simple acute study, probably one could use this individual five or six times. I myself have been used this frequently. It is partly a problem of finding adequate volunteers. If the study continues over many months, then once a year is a maximum. It depends on the study.

*Chairman:* Dr. Smith, I am glad you mentioned Lind. I wonder what an ethical committee would think today of the suggestion that you should inject dairy maids with cowpox and then subject them to contact with smallpox. I think that we may be a shade too timorous.

*Dr. A.J. Fletcher (Syntex):* Dr. Smith, I want to make one point relating to the idea that Phase IV trials should not have any primary marketing aim. I would suggest the corollary that they should not lack marketing aim. Here are two examples. If for good scientific reasons the drug will be marketed with a twice daily dosage regine, in clinical trials there is no point in having a three times daily regime. Secondly, if market research shows that there is no possible reason why a particular indication should be used in the marketing of a drug, is it then ethical to subject patients with this indication to a trial if there is no intention of marketing the drug for that indication?

*Dr. Smith:* You have raised a number of questions. On the first point, I was trying to convey the idea that if the study is effectively carried out, there will be more than sufficient information to provide the marketing department with all the details that they require. Therefore the two aims are really one in this respect. The second point should be satisfied by the mechanics of good clinical research. If not, you are trying to market a drug either for indications or for use in situations for which you have no scientific evidence.

*Dr. J. Domenet (Geigy):* This is a hypothetical question. You have a new anti-inflammatory drug. There are already nine or ten on the market all of which are effective but none are accepted as the best drug. Do you have to do your comparative trials against all of them or do you consult the marketing department to see what their wishes might be?

*Dr. Smith:* There are various ways of tackling this in a practical and pragmatic manner. I think that some pragmatism is helpful in these situations. You can either select a standard drug from one of the nine and compare them or in the final analysis you will probably need, with resources permitting, to compare all of the nine drugs. During the investigation the last four or five may rule themselves out. You are trying to gauge a relationship of safety and toxicity to efficacy. Eventually you may identify a patient population that responds better to your particular drug than any other.

I will make a simple philosophical point. The pundits, who claim that there are a whole series of drugs on the market which all do the same sort of thing. are being too simplistic. There is such wide variation in the human species that it is really a question of identifying the specific patient populations in which each drug works best. I do not think that we are so standard a species that one drug is going to work equally effectively in everybody. In fact we all know that this does not occur.

# PART 2
# SETTING UP CLINICAL TRIALS
(continued)

# 5. Designing the Correct Protocol

D. M. BURLEY

I shall take as my theme the First Book of Kings, Chapter 18, as one of the earlier examples of clinical trial design. To design the correct protocol one needs a methodical approach starting with a question to be answered.

## The question

'How long halt ye between two opinions? If The Lord be God, follow him: but if Baal, then follow him'.

I Kings 18:21

The protocol must set out to frame and answer a question or questions. It is as well to remember Sir Austin Bradford Hill's definition (1971) of a clinical trial: 'A clinical trial is a carefully and ethically designed experiment with the aim of answering some precisely framed question'. Other definitions may include a reference to the use of simultaneous comparisons, or perhaps it should be 'contemporaneous' comparisons. My remarks will concern the comparative type of clinical trial.

Before framing 'the question' one should ask certain questions about the question.
Is it worth answering?
Has it been answered before?
Can it be answered?
Am I the best person to try and answer it?

### Is it worth answering?

It is easy to think up pieces of research and if the subject is sufficiently remote from normal medical practice one can be reasonably sure that it hasn't been explored before. However, as I read the newspapers or my medical journals, I find myself saying more and more often 'this is a question about which I could bear not to know the answer'! Clinical trials take time, trouble, effort and money and involve the goodwill of patients. It is unethical to use these resources unproductively.

### Has it been answered before?

There is a duty to search the medical literature before embarking on a 'new' line of investigation. This literature search will be invaluable when the study is eventually written up, but more importantly it may reveal that the question has already been answered. If the studies and the answer are satisfactory then abandon the project and spare the patients from involvement in a needless experiment. If previous studies have shortcomings, particularly major faults in design, remedy this and point out these shortcomings in the preamble to your protocol, or in the introduction to the paper which is eventually written.

### Can it be answered?

This is often a question of resources. Ensure that the trial can actually be performed by the group involved by asking the questions: Have they the time? Have they the patients? Have they the means to make the necessary measurements? And perhaps most important of all: Have they the skill? You may have to teach them.

### Am I the best person to try and answer it?

This is the humble approach and if carried to extremes you would not do any studies at all. Nevertheless, you would not seek to carry out clinical trials in leprosy in this country, for example, despite good resources in other respects.

Having decided to embark on the study, write down the questions or objectives in language that all can understand and which can be referred to when other problems arise. For example, you may wish to study a new drug (ND) claimed to be of benefit in rheumatoid arthritis.

*Questions.* Is ND superior to a conventional therapy in relieving pain and swelling in classical rheumatoid arthritis?

Are the patients able to state a preference for ND?

Are unwanted effects greater with ND?

It is important to limit the number of questions to be answered since complexity is a constraint in clinical trials. Also, resist attempts to collect 'other interesting information', if this is in any way likely to prejudice the collection of the data essential to answer the main questions. Colleagues often ask 'since you are studying this fascinating group of patients it would be very interesting to administer a questionnaire I have just devised'. Head them off, even if they are senior, unless you feel that the patients can co-operate without influencing the progress of your trial. Sometimes you may judge, in a long trial, that a diversionary game of this kind may sustain interest.

### The Null Hypothesis

THE LORD    ⫢    BAAL

It is customary to assume at the beginning of a trial that there is no difference between two remedies to be compared (or a treatment and a placebo). Therefore, the previously framed questions are put, for statistical purposes, in the form of an hypothesis such as:

'There is no difference between ND and a conventional therapy in relieving pain and swelling in classical rheumatoid arthritis'.

The object of the study is to test this hypothesis. The result will be to accept it or reject it, bearing in mind that rejection can be in two directions in most studies

(ND being superior to conventional therapy or vice versa).

## The patients

Let them, therefore, give us two bullocks...

I Kings 18:23

The most important factors (Burley 1970) which need to be considered when deciding which patients will form the sample to be studied and its corollary the patients to be excluded can be tabulated.

*Factors:*

> Age range
> Sex
> Disease description and severity
> Disease duration
> Previous and current therapy

*Exclusions:*

> Pregnancy (women of childbearing age?)
> Concomitant conditions
> Seriously ill patients
> Danger of drug interaction
> Unco-operative patients.

The greater the constraints placed upon the 'factors' and the longer the list of the 'exclusions', the smaller will be the number of eligible patients. An obvious point, maybe, but who in the industry has not telephoned an investigator who should have been half way through a study only to hear him say 'we have only found two patients of the type you wanted!'?

If you have a list of factors and exclusions it is usually best to produce an entry form of the type shown in Figure 5.1. If all the answers are in the affirmative then the patient is eligible.

## Type of study

> The classical types of study are:
> Comparative groups
> Crossover
> Matched pair
> Sequential

Each of these have their advantages and disadvantages which have been most adequately set out by Maxwell (1969). Crossover studies avoid the need for case matching and stratification, but are unsuitable where the course of the disease is profoundly influenced by the first treatment. Matching pairs is tedious for the investigator and frustrating for the patient who is waiting for his matching partner

ELIGIBILITY FORM*

GROUP : A
FORM  : I

PATIENT'S NAME .........................................................................

HOSPITAL No   .................................................................   TODAY'S DATE ....................................

*tick appropriate box*

|  | | Yes | No |
|---|---|---|---|
| **Is he** | — Male? | ☐ | ☐ |
|  | — Between ages of 35 & 60 years (inclusive)? | ☐ | ☐ |
| **Is there** | — A clinical history of myocardial infarct 2/12 or more ago? | ☐ | ☐ |
|  | — Either a) 2 ECG's available showing typical infarct changes? Or b) If only left bundle branch changes are there also SGOT, CPK or HBD results showing an infarct pattern? | ☐ | ☐ |
| **Have you excluded** | — Cardiogenic shock? | ☐ | ☐ |
|  | — Serious dysrrhythmias? | ☐ | ☐ |
|  | — Heart Failure? | ☐ | ☐ |
|  | — Other cardiac, renal, respiratory or CNS abnormalities, making the patient unsuitable for the study? | ☐ | ☐ |
|  | — Diabetes? | ☐ | ☐ |
|  | — A history of bronchospastic disease (i.e. asthma, chronic bronchitis etc.) contraindicating beta-blockade? | ☐ | ☐ |
| **Can you confirm that** | a) he is not on, or needing, anti-hypertensive drugs? | ☐ | ☐ |
|  | b) he is not taking a tricyclic anti-depressant drug? | ☐ | ☐ |
|  | c) if he is on beta-blockers already, these have not been taken for longer than one month? | ☐ | ☐ |
|  | d) he is fit to return to previous employment, or light work if previously heavy manual labour? | ☐ | ☐ |

*If the answers to all the questions listed above are "YES", then the patient may be eligible for the trial and you should now proceed to fill in the Initial Assessment Form (Form II).
If one of the answers to the questions above is "NO", then the patient must be excluded from the trial.

Fig. 5.1

D953

before he can start his treatment. It is said that comparative group studies involve twice as many patients but halve the trial's duration, whereas crossover studies economise in patients at the expense of time (Fig. 5.2).

**Between groups** (halves time, doubles patients)

| 40 | A |
|----|---|
| 40 | B |

1 month

**Crossover** (halves patients, doubles time)

| 20 | A | B |
|----|---|---|
| 20 | B | A |

1 month          1 month

Fig. 5.2

This is not necessarily true, since it is based on the assumption that all the patients are ready to start at the same time. If it takes 2 months to collect 40 patients the diagram is changed (Fig. 5.3).

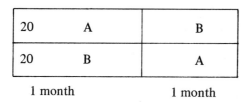

Fig. 5.3

Sequential studies are different and require special charts which look well in publications, but they have lost some of their popularity since they can only answer one simple, albeit important, question at a time. Their merit is that they have stopping rules which may economise in patient numbers at the expense of tighter statistical rules. These have been well described by Armitage (1960) and Bross (1952, 1958).

## Method of allocation of patients to treatments

.......and let them choose one bullock for themselves and cut it in pieces and lay it on wood and put no fire under: I will dress the other bullock and lay it on wood and put no fire under.

I Kings 18:23

It does not say whether a coin was tossed in order to decide which bullock went to one side and which bullock went to the other; but it is essential to employ an efficient method of allocating the patient at random to the treatments *after* their eligibility for the study has been checked. This brings me to the problem of stratification. In other words, what factors do you believe might be important in determining the patients' response to treatment? Will it worry you if chance has decreed a serious imbalance in the distribution of patients with this critical factor as between one treatment and another? Some factors which might be important are:

Patient and his metabolism
Family history
Illness
Other drugs, past or present
Where the patient is treated
Who treats him
Patient's habits and life style

If you are convinced that one or more of these factors is relevant you should stratify the patients, particularly if the numbers are small. Usually a frantic check is made after the trial is over in order to assure the investigators that two groups of patients in a group comparative study are homogeneous. If you do not do this somebody will ask, or worse still, points out the imbalance after publication. If it involves disease severity and nearly all the tough cases were on your favoured drug you are almost bound to be disappointed with the answer. The stratification procedure involves having separate randomisation lists for each sub group of patients (Fig. 5.4).

| List A | | List B | |
|---|---|---|---|
| Acute (Active) | | Chronic (Inactive) | |
| 1. ........................... | X | 21. ........................... | Y |
| 2. ........................... | X | 22. ........................... | X |
| 3. ........................... | Y | 23. ........................... | X |
| 4. ........................... | X | 24. ........................... | Y |
| 5. ........................... | Y | 25. ........................... | Y |
| ........................... | | ........................... | |
| ........................... | | ........................... | |
| ........................... | | ........................... | |

Fig. 5.4

The greater number of stratifications and the more levels chosen multiplies the number of ramdomisation lists, for instance:

|  |  |
|---|---|
| SEX | MALE/FEMALE |
| SEVERITY | ACUTE/INTERMEDIATE/CHRONIC |
| 2 x 3 | 6 LISTS |

Theoretically it is possible to have a very large number of stratifications. Taves (1974) indicated a method of carrying out such stratification, even if it meant that some cells in the chart had zero or only one patient in them. There are other methods, but this is not the place to go into them. I would only say that they require expertise, data handling equipment and first class communication between the investigator, the pharmacy, the statistician and the drug company. How often do you get that?

## Numbers

Obtain statistical advice during the planning stage of any clinical trial, in particular to decide on the number of patients that will be required to accept or reject the null hypothesis at an appropriate significance level. The objectives are:

To avoid accepting a treatment which is of no value ($\alpha$)

To avoid rejecting a treatment which is of value ($\beta$)

To decide on the size of the difference in activity between two drugs which one hopes to detect ($\theta$)

The key to all this is numbers. Charts and tables have been constructed to help with this, notably those by Clark and Downie (1966) and Maxwell (1968).

## Measurement

And call ye on the name of your gods and I will call on the name of the Lord and the God that answereth by fire, let him be God.

I Kings 18:24

Detailed consideration of measurements and their validity will be covered in later chapters. There are essentially three types of measurement:

Nominal

Ordinal

Interval

The first and the last are the most commonly used. Subjective measurements are usually nominal; some psychiatric rating scales being notable exceptions. Objective measurements are usually on interval scales. Beware of the following:

Inter and intra observer error

Digit preference

Lack of sensitivity of some nominal scales

Incorrect analysis of rating scales

Crombie (1963) pointed out many years ago the desirability of having nominal scales of 5 or 6 points, provided the terms used were clear.

## Bias

And they cried aloud, and cut themselves, after their manner, with knives and lancets, till the blood gushed out upon them.

I Kings 18:28

Bias is to be avoided and may occur at different stages of a clinical trial. Bias may occur at the time of selection of patients. This is avoided by random allocation of treatments to patients, *after* the patient has entered the trial. At a later stage bias may occur, particularly if subjective measurements are being made, because of enthusiasm for one or other of the treatments on the part of the investigator or patient. Matching drugs and matching placebos have been devised to avoid this, but 'code cracking' is an amusing game and is all too easy in many trials. Recent analysis of 'matching preparations' by Hill, Nunn and Wallace Fox (1976), has revealed many shortcomings and I would remind you of the recommendations of Joyce (1968) (Table 5.1).

Table 5.1  Minimal specifications to manufacturers of capsules or tablets to be used in a comparative trial

| 1. To match perfectly* for: | 2. To match as closely as possible for: |
| --- | --- |
| a. Shape | a. Taste on licking |
| b. Size | b. Taste on chewing |
| c. Surface colour | c. Internal colour |
| d. Surface texture | d. Internal texture |
| e. Weight | e. Smell |
| | f. Specific gravity |

3.  To bear no external distinguishing signs, and to be put up in containers free of identifying marks. The containers for each treatment should be packed in separate boxes labelled with the identity of their contents.

* Samples must be indistinguishable to a panel of four judges.

However, it should not be necessary to carry out a trial of 'placebo spotting' which is more complicated than the trial proper, and there are also other ways of achieving blindness (Crombie, 1976). I would add to the Joyce table the additional point that tablets may change colour during the course of a trial. White tablets frequently go off-white or yellow, but their 'matching' placebos do not necessarily change.

Placebo reactions have a diluting effect on the results of a trial and it is not always recognised that these may be positive or negative. These ideas are illustrated in Figures 5.5 to 5.7. In Figure 5.5 the drug effect is 20 units for drug A and 10 units for drug B, a 2 : 1 difference. This will be harder to detect if there are 40 units of

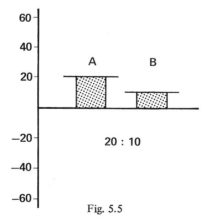

Fig. 5.5

placebo effect due to investigator enthusiasm. Now the ratio is 6 : 5 as in Figure 5.6. Investigator pessimism may produce a negative placebo effect of 40 units. Now the situation is not quite so bad, since the measurable difference will be - 2 : -3, but the diluting effect will still be greater than if there had been no placebo effect to consider (Figure 5.7).

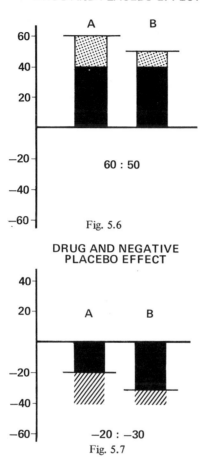

DRUG AND PLACEBO EFFECT

60 : 50

Fig. 5.6

DRUG AND NEGATIVE PLACEBO EFFECT

−20 : −30

Fig. 5.7

### Drug administration

This becomes most complicated when oral treatments need to be compared with parenteral treatments and when variable dosage schemes are used. The former problem is met by double dummy techniques (Figure 5.8) and the latter by individual daily or weekly packaging schemes. The following scheme allowed three drugs to be used in a crossover trial, all of which were used at different dosage levels (Figure 5.9 and Table 5.2).

The daily packages contained one to four capsules per slot to be taken three times daily. Hence, dosage could be increased from one capsule t.d.s. to four capsules t.d.s. according to the patient's response. Three drugs were in use in a crossover design and Table 5.2 sets out the number of active and placebo capsules used in order to achieve different ranges of dosage either twice or three times daily. Remember, however, that such ingeneous arrangements involve many staff hours of packaging and may be yet another factor delaying the start of the trial.

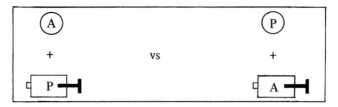

Fig. 5.8 Double dummy. Half the patients receive an active tablet and a dummy injection, the other half a dummy tablet and an active injection.

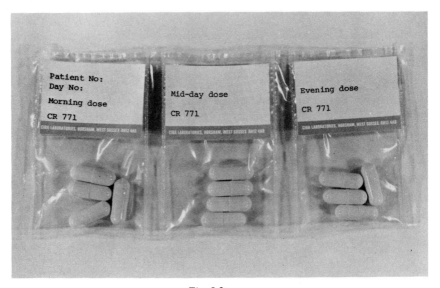

Fig. 5.9

### Adverse reactions

These are best classified into three groups as my colleague Dr. Forrest (1973, 1975) does in his many multicentre studies.

Trivial reactions, nuisance value

Mild reactions, of importance for comparative purposes but not causing discontinuance of treatment

Serious reactions, leading to discontinuance of therapy.

Table 5.2  Drug dosage and increments

| 80mg oxprenolol | 250mg methyldopa | 100mg spironolactone | | | | | |
|---|---|---|---|---|---|---|---|
| | | Drug | | | Placebo | | |
| | | M | N | N | M | N | N |
| **Oxprenolol (80mg)** | | | | | | | |
| 160 mg - 1 tds | | 1 | 0 | 1 | 0 | 1 | 0 |
| 320 mg - 2 tds | | 2 | 1 | 1 | 0 | 1 | 1 |
| 450 mg - 3 tds | | 2 | 2 | 2 | 1 | 1 | 1 |
| 640 mg - 4 tds | | 3 | 2 | 3 | 1 | 2 | 1 |
| **Methyldopa (150mg)** | | | | | | | |
| 750 mg - 1 tds | | 1 | 1 | 1 | 0 | 0 | 0 |
| 1500 mg - 2 tds | | 2 | 2 | 2 | 0 | 0 | 0 |
| 2250 mg - 3 tds | | 3 | 3 | 3 | 0 | 0 | 0 |
| 3000 mg - 4 tds | | 4 | 4 | 4 | 0 | 0 | 0 |
| **Spironolactone (100mg)** | | | | | | | |
| 300 mg - 1 tds | | 1 | 1 | ? | 0 | 0 | 0 |
| 300 mg - 2 tds | | 1 | 1 | 1 | 1 | 1 | 1 |
| 300 mg - 3 tds | | 1 | 1 | 1 | 2 | 2 | 2 |
| 300 mg - 4 tds | | 1 | 1 | 1 | 3 | 3 | 3 |

M=morning, N=noon, N=night

It is also important to distinguish those reactions which are part and parcel of the drug's action and those which are unexpected (idiosyncratic). Defaulting is linked with adverse reactions. Provision must be made in any trial protocol to follow up a patient who fails to attend at an expected time. There may be a simple explanation, but he may have defaulted because he is ill or thinks one of the drugs is making him ill. A home visit may be essential if the patient cannot be contacted in any other way.

Defaulting patients may be, and patients removed because of side effects invariably are, relevant factors in the analysis of clinical trial results. It is only in special trial plans involving for instance a factorial design that drop-outs are legitimately replaced. Finally, bear in mind that legal provisions govern the reporting of adverse reactions in clinical trials. These vary from country to country and will save a lot of pain if correct forms are obtained and filled in. It is extremely difficult to acquire the data after the reaction is over.

## Results

The analysis of the results will be tackled later in this book, but you may like to be reminded of the results in our biblical trial.

### Positive result

Hear me, O Lord, hear me, that this people may know thou art The Lord God... then the fire of The Lord fell, and consumed the burnt sacrifice...

I Kings 18:37

*Negative result*

They called on the name of Baal from morning even until noon, saying O Baal, hear us. But there was no voice, nor any that answered.

I Kings 18:26

## Summary

The correct protocol design can be summarised under the following main headings:

*Objectives* - QUESTIONS
*Material* - PATIENTS
*Trial design* - numbers
*Treatments* - allocation - placebos
*Measurements*
*Adverse reactions* - drop outs

and these subsidiary headings:

*Record forms* - printing
*Drug presentation* - matching
*Logistics* - record keeping - drug quantities
*Report writing (publication)* - literature search

## General comments

Having summarised the important ingredients of correct protocol design, there are a few ancillary points to be considered and which should be commented on at the end of the protocol. These are:

Ethics and compensation
Cost of trial (estimated)
Time scale
Have you a Clinical Trial Certificate?

It is usual now for hospitals to have Ethics Committees to which protocols are submitted. They will consider not only the ethics of the drug administration but also the risks attendant upon the various investigations to be carried out, which will yield the measurement data. The question of compensation for injury during a clinical trial is controversial and outside the scope of this chapter. Costs of trials are constantly escalating and the likely support costs in terms of staff time, equipment and materials will need to be worked out beforehand and apportioned. A realistic time score should be drawn up with correct allowance being made for preparation of materials, collection of patients, drug treatment and washout periods. Finally, you should check that a valid Clinical Trial Certificate is held to cover the study or the indication for which a medication is to be prescribed. The onus falls on the pharmaceutical company whenever they are making supplies of drugs or placebos available to an investigator for clinical trial purposes.

However, if I was to leave only one message, I would council simplicity. Our biblical trial asked one simple question, involved two subjects, one measurement, took some six hours to complete and the answer had a profound effect on the destiny of the Children of Israel.

THE LORD $>$ BAAL

## REFERENCES

Armitage, P. (1960) *Sequential Medical Trials*. Blackwell, Oxford. pp. 15-24.

Bross, I. (1952) Sequential medical plans. *Biometrics*. 8, 188-205.

Bross, I. (1958) Sequential medical trials. *J. Chron. Dis.* 8, 349.

Burley, D.M. (1970) Preliminary design - the ideal clinical trial. In *The Principles and Practice of Clinical Trials*. Ed. Harris and Fitzgerald. E. & S. Livingstone, Edinburgh.

Clark, C.J. & Downie, C.C. (1966) A method for the rapid determination of the number of patients to include in a controlled clinical trial. *Lancet* ii, 1357.

Cromie, B.W. (1963) The feet of clay of the double blind trial. *Lancet*, ii, 994.

Cromie, B.W. (1976) 'Not so double-blind'. *Brit. med. J.* i, 710.

First Book of Kings, Chapter 18, verses 21, 23, 24, 26, 28 and 37.

Forrest, W.A. (1973): Subjective comparison between oxprenolol (Trasicor) and long-acting nitrates in the treatment of angina pectoris in general practice. *J. Int. Med. Res.* i, 253.

Forrest W.A. (1975) A comparison between daily and nightly dose regimen of amitriptyline and maprotiline (Ludiomil) in the treatment of reactive depression in general practice. *J. Int. Med. Res.* 3, Suppl. 2, 120.

Hill, A.B. (1971) *Principles of Medical Statistics*. 2nd. ed., p.273.

Hill, L.E., Nunn, A.J. & Wallace Fox (1976) Matching quality of agents employed in double blind controlled clinical trials. *Lancet* i, 352.

Joyce, C.R.B. (1968) Psychopharmacology: dimensions and perspectives. In *Mind and Medicine Monographs*, pp. 215-242. Tavistock Publications.

Maxwell, C. (1968) The significance of significance. *Clin. Trial.* 5, 1015.

Maxwell, C. (1969) *Clinical Trials' Protocol - A Primer for Clinical Trials*. Stuart Phillips Publications.

Taves, D.R. (1974) Minimization: A new method of assigning patients to treatment and control groups. *Clin. Pharmacol. Ther.* 15, 5, 443.

# 6.  Designing the Report Form

F. GRADY

In 1975, McLean, Foote and Wagner published a bibliography of manual, automated and computer based techniques. This list covered the collection and processing of medical history data and comprised 720 separate references to the literature of the last 30 years. In the current issue of the same journal, Mellner, Selander and Welodarski (1976) describe some of the difficulties in the use of the questionnaire method for medical history taking.

Extensive work has already been completed in this area and more is still going on. Much of the bibliography refers to systems which require a total commitment to the particular procedures required. That may be perfect for certain aspects of medical history taking. It was considered at ICI Pharmaceuticals Division that although the data acquisition procedures demanded for clinical trials were in many ways equivalent to the demands of medical history taking, there were other factors which contraindicated rigid alignment with any precise system.

It was considered that the objective of a clinical trial was to demonstrate as clearly and as quickly as possible the efficacy and the safety of a drug in humans and that data acquisition had to be in such a manner as to meet this objective. Unfortunately, this objective referred to a clinical trial  in singular. Our situation required a system which would cater for any number of trials of any numbers of drugs in all areas of application. When considering how best to meet this situation, in house knowledge of the handling of clinical trial data was compared to a formal study carried out by Blackeney-Edwards, Eddins and Rhodes (1970) of John Hoskyns and Co. Ltd. These deliberations led to the present system our group uses to handle data arising from clinical and animal field trials. This system is best described as a 'Non-System'. It relies in its entirety on four items: the clinical trial report form, the punched card, and two commercially available ICL(software) packages, FIND-2 (*File Interrogation Nineteen Hundred*) and SURVEY ANALYSIS.

In considering how to meet the problem of data acquisition in clinical trials, we came to the conclusion that the more we defined a system for any single clinical trial or similar group of trials, the less likely we were to be able to use that system for other trials. Taking this a step further we rationalised that even had we designed a system which encompassed all the trials we had handled in the past (since 1962) and extrapolated as much as we could into the future, we would still not have a system sufficiently robust to carry us through the next five to ten years. Therefore, we moved away from the defined system towards a philosophy of maximum flexibility and minimum constraints. We decided, on our experience with clinical trial data and our knowledge of the capacity and flexibility of the softward packages, that subject to the data being recorded within the normal limits of machine acceptable conventions, then we would be able to handle all the trials with which we were presented. This allowed the clinician to be unconstrained at the trial design stage, with classification, analysis and evaluation being carried out within the capacity of the packages. So far, our faith in our 'Non-System' has been justified. We are currently handling something in excess of 120 clinical trials of all shapes, volumes, colours and sizes. These range from large numbers of records with large amounts of data, for example a 30,000 record B-blockade study, to small numbers of patients with vast amounts of data, such as 20 patient dental studies. Each patient has 32 teeth (spaces are included), each tooth has five surfaces, each surface has several facets, each facet has several grades, each patient is examined several times. One study of 20 patients created a punched card record file of over 8,000 cards which we reckoned were the equivalent of almost 50,000 subrecords. The list of possible applications seems endless.

The system is equally suitable for all types of trial: Latin Square, single blind, double blind, with and without crossovers, with and without washout periods, single centre, multicentre, or for open studies not aligned with trials of drugs. The system is readily useable in all countries irrespective of language differences. We have worked on over 200 clinical and field trials covering all the ICI pharmaceutical products in a large number of applications. As yet we have found no areas of clinical trial work where our basic approach of a non aligned data collection record cannot be applied.

Our system basically consists of a record sheet (or more often a series of record sheets) completed by the clinician. The completed records and sent to the Division where a manual intellectual edit is carried out. This edit is valuable at the start of the trial to ensure that there is no misinterpretation of the questionnaire particularly in multicentre trials where the large number of people involved increases the potential for different interpretations of questions. This edit also highlights missing data and the taking of both options in a mutually exclusive question, for instance, Alive, Yes; Dead, Yes. 'Nonsense' answers such as age at menopause for men, weights given in kilos instead of pounds and vice versa, dates of onset of disease preceeding date of birth and patient visits following patient death. Any queries are resolved with the clinician, and with his agreement the necessary amendments are made to the records. Where data is missing, the relevant record field is coded to identify it as missing data and to deal with it appropriately in distribution counts, correlations and calculations. The amended forms are key punched into cards using a commercial bureau, the cards are read to file initially in a card image format and reformatted for use with the two software packages as appropriate. Data validation is carried out and amended data updated onto the file. Updates usually consist of additional sequential visit data being added to the end of the file. At the completion of the data acquisition stage, the original clinical trial records are microfilmed and then held in deep store. Access to the records is initially via a microfilm reader, reducing the necessity to retrieve originals to a minimum. The punched card records complete their function as a data input medium and are retained as a security record for several years after the end of the trial. The original records received from the clinician, the microfilm copy of these records and the magnetic tape of card images are retained indefinitely. All retrieval, interrogation, classification, correlations and distributions are carried out using the FIND-2 and SURVEY ANALYSIS packages.

The strength and weakness of the system lie in the design of the patient record form. We selected a questionnaire style report form for data acquisition because it is suitable for use in all environments. There are other alternatives such as direct data entry systems and video display units, but these can not be used in all trials and in all areas. The form has many attractions. It is cheap to produce. An A4 size report form prepared from final draft manuscript, would cost £20 to £30 for artwork and typesetting depending on the complexity of the record. Printing costs vary with size of batch required, but duplicate or triplicate forms work out at 2 to 3p per sheet for runs of 1,000. The form is easy to use, most people accept form filling as part of everyday life and another form for completion presents no special problems. The use of No Carbon Required (NCR) pressure sensitive paper in duplicate or triplicate record sets coupled with accurate printing registration permits several copies to be made simultaneously. This allows the original to be despatched to us, a second copy to be held in the patient's total notes whilst a third could be held separately by the investigator. Use of a form permits maximum flexibility in shape, size and colour. Our current sizes range from small cards suitable for inclusion in a patient's National Health Service folder in general practice through the great majority of A4 size to the extreme of a 20 page booklet for the New Zealand Farm Survey. Different colours of paper and printing are useful for visual identification of record types in the clinics. In an average trial four types of record would be entry, visit, biochemistry and trial termination records in which case different coloured paper may be used for each type, or alternatively the same colour of paper overprinted in four different coloured inks.

The form must itself fulfill three distinct and separate functions. In chronological order of use, it must allow the clinician to record the data pertinent to that patient in that particular trial, it must serve as a punching document to the key punch operator in a non-medical situation and it must ensure that when all the records have been fed to the computer they are correctly designated and correctly related to each other.

In form design these functions occur in reverse order and the final item covers two different types of data management. The first type is information containing the structure of the record relevant to its function and relative to data relationships within the punched cards and hence the computer. This is best demonstrated by using as an example one of our clinical trials in intermittent claudication (Fig. 6.1). The data acquisition requirements for the trial called for an extensive history record; a series of visit records to be completed at entry and at each two month visit, with extra data arising from a more extensive examination at entry and at each six month visit; a biochemistry form to record the data which had resulted in the selection of the patient for trial and the six monthly measurements; and finally a trial termination form which summarised certain items at the end of the trial.

The information needed to structure this set of records was:

| | |
|---|---|
| History | Type O |
| Visit | Type 1 |
| Biochemistry Screening | Type 2 |
| Biochemistry Therapy | Type 3 |
| Termination | Type 4 |

Within the history record there are three subsections referring to the patient in general,

ICI Use only    Col. 1
D □ 1
P □ 2

IMPERIAL CHEMICAL INDUSTRIES — PHARMACEUTICALS DIVISION
**DOUBLE BLIND TRIAL OF CLOFIBRATE IN INTERMITTENT CLAUDICATION**

Hospital No. □ 2

VISIT RECORD (Complete at all visits including entry)

Patient Name _____    Patient trial No. □□ 3 4    Sheet □ 1 8    Record □ 1 9    Date □□□□□□ 10 11 12 13 14 15    Months on trial □□ 16 17

(Code 00 at entry)

| Activity 18 | | Restrictions due to 19 | | CURRENT STATUS | Angina 20 | | New infarct 22 | |
|---|---|---|---|---|---|---|---|---|
| Normal | 1 | Coronary Dis | 1 | | Yes | 1 | Yes | 1 |
| Restricted | 2 | Claudication | 2 | | No | 2 | No | 2 |
| Tot. Incap. | 3 | Cerebovasc. Dis | 3 | | Angina of effort 21 | | Weight | |
| | | Amputation | 4 | | On severe exertion | 1 | 23 24 25 | |
| | | Arthritis | 5 | | On walking | 2 | □□□ Kgs | |
| | | Other | 6 | | At rest | 3 | | |

| CVA 26 | | None vasc. operation since last visit 28 | | Smoking (per day) 29 | | Therapy 30 | | Specify other |
|---|---|---|---|---|---|---|---|---|
| Yes | 1 | Yes | 1 | None | 1 | Digitalis | 1 | _____ |
| No | 2 | No | 2 | <10 | 2 | β-Blockers | 2 | _____ |
| 27 | | Specify | | 11—20 | 3 | Vasodilators | 3 | _____ |
| Worsened | 1 | _____ | | >20 | 4 | Fat reduced diet | 4 | _____ |
| Unchanged | 2 | _____ | | Pipe | 5 | Others | 5 | _____ |
| Improved | 3 | _____ | | Cigars | 6 | | | _____ |

**CLAUDICATION**

RIGHT SIDE — (Punch Operator, new card, repunch col. 1—4, 8, col. 9/2 10—17 incl.)
Distance walked (leave blank if stopped due to other leg)

| 18 19 20 21 | | Claudication Site 23 | | Progress since started treatment (leave blank at initial visit) 24 | |
|---|---|---|---|---|---|
| □□□□ yds. | | None | 0 | | |
| Stopped due to 22 | | Thigh | 1 | Worsened | 1 |
| claudication  No | 0 | Buttock | 2 | Unchanged | 2 |
| in this leg  Yes | 1 | Calf | 3 | Improved | 3 |
| Other causes | 2 | | | | |

LEFT SIDE — (Punch Operator, new card, repunch col. 1—4, 8, col. 9/3 10—17 incl.)
Distance walked (leave blank if stopped due to other leg)

| 18 19 20 21 | | Claudication Site 23 | | Progress since started treatment (leave blank at initial visit) 24 | |
|---|---|---|---|---|---|
| □□□□ yds. | | None | 0 | | |
| Stopped due to 22 | | Thigh | 1 | Worsened | 1 |
| claudication  No | 0 | Buttock | 2 | Unchanged | 2 |
| in this leg  Yes | 1 | Calf | 3 | Improved | 3 |
| Other causes | 2 | | | | |

**PULSES**

| Femoral 25 | | Popliteal 26 | | Ant. tib. 27 | | Post tib. 28 | | Femoral 25 | | Popliteal 26 | | Ant. tib. 27 | | Post. tib. 28 | |
|---|---|---|---|---|---|---|---|---|---|---|---|---|---|---|---|
| Normal | 1 | Normal | 1 | Normal | 1 | Normal | 1 | Normal | 1 | Normal | 1 | Normal | 1 | Normal | 1 |
| Diminished | 2 | Diminished | 2 | Diminished | 2 | Diminished | 2 | Diminished | 2 | Diminished | 2 | Diminished | 2 | Diminished | 2 |
| Absent | 3 | Absent | 3 | Absent | 3 | Absent | 3 | Absent | 3 | Absent | 3 | Absent | 3 | Absent | 3 |

| REST PAIN | | VASCULAR OPERATION 31 Specify | | REST PAIN | | VASCULAR OPERATION 31 Specify | |
|---|---|---|---|---|---|---|---|
| 29 Progress since started treatment | | | | 29 Progress since started treatment | | | |
| Yes | 1 | Yes | 1 | Yes | 1 | Yes | 1 |
| No | 2 | No | 2 | No | 2 | No | 2 |
| 30 | | Date | | 30 | | Date | |
| Worsened | 1 | 32 33 34 35 36 37 | | Worsened | 1 | 32 33 34 35 36 37 | |
| Unchanged | 2 | □□□□□□ | | Unchanged | 2 | □□□□□□ | |
| Improved | 3 | | | Improved | 3 | | |

| ULCERS 38 | | GANGRENE/TROPHIC 40 | | ULCERS 38 | | GANGRENE/TROPHIC 40 | |
|---|---|---|---|---|---|---|---|
| Progress since started treatment | | Progress since started treatment | | Progress since started treatment | | Progress since started treatment | |
| Yes | 1 | Yes | 1 | Yes | 1 | Yes | 1 |
| No | 2 | No | 2 | No | 2 | No | 2 |
| 39 | | 41 | | 39 | | 41 | |
| Worsened | 1 | Worsened | 1 | Worsened | 1 | Worsened | 1 |
| Unchanged | 2 | Unchanged | 2 | Unchanged | 2 | Unchanged | 2 |
| Improved | 3 | Improved | 3 | Improved | 3 | Improved | 3 |

**BLOOD PRESSURE GRADIENT** (Only at 00, 06, 12 mths. etc.)

| RESTING | Arm 42 43 44 | Foot 48 49 50 | Difference 51 52 | Claudication Count 53 54 55 56 | RESTING | Arm 43 43 44 | Foot 48 49 50 | Difference 51 52 | Claudication Count 53 54 55 56 |
|---|---|---|---|---|---|---|---|---|---|
| Sys. | □□□ | □□□ | □□ | □□ □□ | Sys. | □□□ | □□□ | □□ | □□ □□ |
| Dia. | 45 46 47 □□□ | | | mins  secs | Dia. | 45 46 47 □□□ | | | mins  secs |

| AFTER EXERCISE | | 58 59 60 | 64 65 66 | 67 68 | Time 69 70 at min □□ min pressure | AFTER EXERCISE | | 58 59 60 | 64 65 66 | 67 68 | Time 69 70 at min □□ min pressure |
|---|---|---|---|---|---|---|---|---|---|---|---|
| /1 sec | 1 | Sys. □□□ | □□□ | □□ | 71 72 | /1 sec | 1 | Sys. □□□ | □□□ | □□ | 71 72 |
| /5 sec | 2 | 61 62 63 Dia. □□□ | minimum pressure | to return to prev. value □□ min | | /5 sec | 2 | 61 62 63 Dia. □□□ | minimum pressure | to return to prev. value □□ min | |

(Punch Operator End 9/3 card here.)

| TRIAL STATE 73 | | If withdrawn due to 74 | | COMMENTS (including comments on withdrawals) 75 | |
|---|---|---|---|---|---|
| Continuing | | Cardiovasc.death | 1 | Yes | 1 |
| Withdrawn | 2 | Other death | 2 | No | 2 |
| Lost to trial | 3 | Other causes | 3 | | |

Signature _____ Date _____

Fig. 6.1

to the right side and to the left side of the body. Accordingly, the history record structure becomes:

    0  :  1
    0  :  2
    0  :  3

The visit record must be identifiable and also classifiable by its visit sequence. In this particular case the actual month number rather than the sequential visit number is included in order to retrieve separately these records at 00, 06, 12 and 18 months which contain extra clinical data. Again the record requires three subsections to accommodate general, right side and left side information. The visit record becomes:

| Type | Subsection | Month on trial |
|------|------------|----------------|
| 1 | 1 | 00 |
| 1 | 2 | 00 |
| 1 | 3 | 00 |
| 1 | 1 | 02 |
| 1 | 2 | 02 |
| 1 | 3 | 02 |
| ↓ | ↓ | ↓ |
| 1 | 1 | 18 |
| 1 | 2 | 18 |
| 1 | 3 | 18 |

The biochemistry comprises a preliminary screening record and a sequence of identical biochemical records which must be linked to the six-monthly visit records at which the blood samples were taken. Since all the biochemistry for the whole of the trial is contained as perforated subsections on one single record form, each subsection was separately designated. The biochemistry record becomes:

*For the screening test:*

    2    1    99        99 is used as a code to differentiate from
                        00 entry data

*For the visit related data:*

    3    1    00
    3    2    06
    3    3    12
    3    4    18

The trial termination record serves a dual purpose. It gives the clinician an opportunity for summary or global assessment and it rounds off the records of the patient in the trial and establishes the fact that the patient has reached a precise end point. The record shows simply:

| Type | Months on trial to termination |
|------|-------------------------------|
| 4 | 06, 10, 16, etc. |

This type of record structuring gives complete flexibility in the subsequent manipulation of records. It gives the facility to retrieve and bring together any combination of the records: it is possible to compare all the 06 month data with the 12 and the 18 to establish time required to observe improvement; to look at the 06 month biochemical changes and compare them with the clinical picture at 06 months, 10 months and 12 months to establish if the changes in the biochemistry are indications of subsequent clinical changes; to look at global assessment in the termination record and relate it to duration of disease or age of onset of disease recorded in the history record. Precise structuring of the records creates maximum flexibility.

The second type of management function is that concerned with the operation of the trial. This would normally include a trial centre designation, patient record number, possibly coded patient initials, dates of visits, current therapy, tablet counts and bottle exchange as appropriate. Data of this type enable a close control to be kept over the progress of the trial permitting such questions as: 'How many patient months have been covered at each of the trial centres?' or 'Has this particular patient turned up for her six month visit?' In staggered entry trials with patients not in a uniform cycle, it allows us to find, for example, all the patients who should have turned up for their ten month visit and have not done so.

The second function of the record is related specifically to the computer aspect of trial handling. The record must provide the means of communication to the key punch operator to ensure high accuracy in punched card preparation and ultimately high accuracy of data in the computer. The record must present clearly to the key punch operator what is required. We attempt to do this in the majority of our trials by printing card punching instructions, punched card column and row numbers on the form itself, thus creating a direct punching document. We prefer this method and find that it is acceptable to the most clinicians and least troublesome to the key punch operators. The alternative method, which we use when the numbers and punching instructions are not desired, is to leave out the numbers completely or insert only numbers at the start and the end of sections and then to supply either a detailed punching instruction or a transparent mask to the operators. Both these procedures reduce accuracy and speed in card preparation. We avoid them where possible.

The third function of the record is to permit the clinician to record his data in a manner that is most meaningful to him and to the objectives of the trial. To help him realise these objectives he is offered almost unlimited facilities in the design of the form. Data may be represented in punched card format in several different ways. Most of our trials use a combination of methods, although the clinician is probably not aware that he is using different techniques. The commonest way of representing data is standard alphanumeric where the word or number is represented in the card. This allows text entry, such as patient name or initials, it allows data entry, for instance, 12.08.75 or direct numerical values, blood pressure 120/80. Another technique is to use a column of a card as a concept and then ask the binary question 'Previous History of Heart Disease' Yes/No. A third technique is to group together adjacent areas of data and allocate a joint designation. For example, age might be encoded as 20-29=2, 30-39=3, 40-49=4, etc. This presents a simple way to record data, but can also present difficulties in analysis and evaluation if statistical comparison of age is required. Data must always be put in with a view to retrieval. One further technique of data representation valuable in descriptive or soft data areas is the use of multipunching. This will allow any number of preset arbitrary terms to be used in recording a description of any item. We have used this effectively in recording ECG information where a comparatively large number of descriptors may be set up, with any combination from none to all being used. The multipunch machine is a special facility not generally available.

The clinician has complete control over what form the data will take within the records for his own trial. Since each record form is designed individually and since each trial is held separately in the computer system, there is no impingement of trials upon each other. This gives each clinician full autonomy in deciding upon the content of his record sheet. Also within his direct control is whether he wishes to have a separate record for each patient visit or have a single record covering all the visits (Fig. 6.2). The questions are those requested by the clinician, but advice is usually given on the precise wording with a view to asking completely unambigous questions in the most succint manner.

Using current trials we have made a simple survey of how clinicians have used patient record design facilities. Over 60 per cent are run on a conventional approach and have basic similarities, although all are designed and operated as completely separate studies. In this 60 per cent, records consist of routine data collection of name, trial number, sex, weight, date of visit, linked to the following sections; medical history, covering concurrent disease, previous therapy, smoking habits, concurrent therapy; current clinical assessment to ascertain the state of the patient at commencement of the trial and provide the baseline against which the patient will be compared at each visit; a corresponding laboratory record to provide baseline biochemistry or haematology against which visit laboratory data will be compared; and finally the trial termination record.

The design of remaining trials has created a variety of form usage. The following examples give some indication of possible applications. In trials of products in allergic rhinitis and bronchial asthma the large amount of variation in patient condition allied to the practical difficulties of bringing the patient to the clinic more frequently than once a week lead to the design of a patient 'Do it Yourself' recording form (Fig. 6.3). This is designed to assess frequency and severity of symptoms based on the patient's own assessment. The assessment is subjective, but has the advantage that it does not require long term symptom recall by the patient. Recurrent aphthous ulceration presented problems in location, identification, patient memory and severity. Figure 6.4 shows a record designed to overcome these problems. At the commencement of the trial the patient locates all the ulcers present, labels them A, B, C, etc. and writes the letters on the facial diagram. On each subsequent day he grades the ulcers present using the severity code and adds any new ulcers to the record. This appeared to be the only way in which we could collect trial data of this type directly from the patient. Dental studies present their own peculiar problems. Large amounts of almost identical data require very careful designation.

Long term trials require special attention to the physical volume of the records especially where the study is carried out in general practice with limited storage space. Figures 6.5 and 6.6 show a two part record designed to cover initial registration and allow for a simple 10 year follow up of blood pressure and therapy. Simple instructions may be given by printing on the reverse of the card (Fig. 6.7 and 6.8). We are convinced that this type of questionnaire record provides the best system for clinical trial data acquisition. There are problems. Three which we meet most frequently are additional information, side effects and comparative questions.

IMPERIAL CHEMICAL INDUSTRIES LTD. PHARMACEUTICALS DIVISION
TRIAL OF VIVALAN IN OBESE DEPRESSIVES. DR. MATHUR, BILLINGE HOSPITAL

Patient's Initials        Patient No.

Age        Sex M / F        Smoking Habits — Nil / Mod. / Heavy

Diagnosis ......

ICI Use Only

HAMILTON RATING SCALE FOR DEPRESSION

| Item No. | 1 | 2 | 3 | 4 | 5 | 6 | 7 | 8 | 9 | 10 | 11 | 12 | 13 | 14 | 15 | 16 | 17 | 18 | 19 | 20 | 21 |
|---|---|---|---|---|---|---|---|---|---|---|---|---|---|---|---|---|---|---|---|---|---|

Item labels: Depressed Mood, Guilt, Suicide, Insomnia — early, Insomnia — middle, Insomnia — late, Work & Interests, Retardation, Agitation, Anxiety — psychic, Anxiety — somatic, Somatic symptoms — G.I., Somatic symptoms — gen., Genital symptoms, Hypochondriasis, Loss of weight, Insight, Diurnal variation, Depersonalisation & Derealisation, Paranoid symptoms, Obsessional

Score as HRSD on Reverse

* Col. 7/8 — Entry (00), 2 Weeks (02), 4 Weeks (04), 8 Weeks (08), 12 Weeks (12)

↑ Global assessment scoring
0 – Absent
1 – Minimal
2 – Mild
3 – Moderate
4 – Severe
5 – Intolerable

Pulse Rate 30 31 32
B.P. Syst. 33 34 35    Diast. 36 37 38
Wakefield self-assessment scale 39 40
Global assessment 41 ↑
Linear Hunger scale mm. 42 43
Skin Fold Thickness mms (Average of both sides)
Triceps 44 45 46 47
Subscapular 48 49 50 51
Weight Kg (To 1st Decimal) 52 53 54 55

Side Effects        56/1 56/2 Yes No
2nd Visit (2nd wk)
3rd Visit (4th wk)
4th Visit (8th wk)
5th Visit (12th wk)

If yes, specify ......

Withdrawals   Reason and date ......

Signed as correct ......        Date ......

*Repeat Cols. 1—6

Fig. 6.2

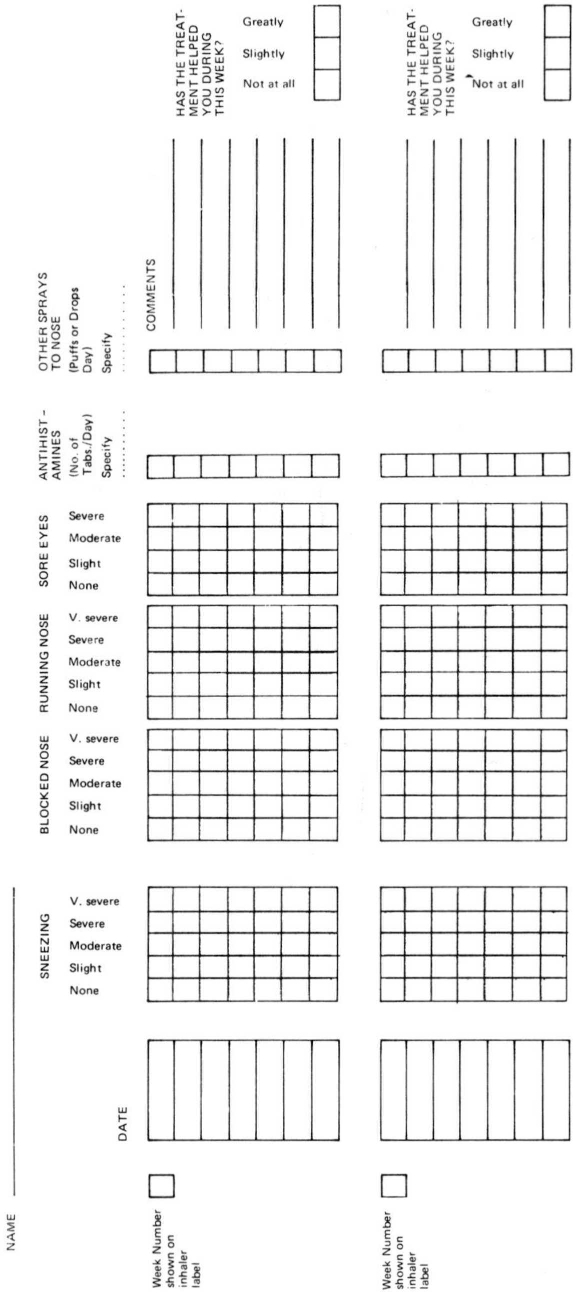
NAME
Week Number shown on inhaler label
DATE
SNEEZING
V. severe
Severe
Moderate
Slight
None
BLOCKED NOSE
V. severe
Severe
Moderate
Slight
None
RUNNING NOSE
V. severe
Severe
Moderate
Slight
None
SORE EYES
Severe
Moderate
Slight
None
ANTIHIST - AMINES (No. of Tabs./Day) Specify
OTHER SPRAYS TO NOSE (Puffs or Drops Day) Specify
COMMENTS
HAS THE TREAT- MENT HELPED YOU DURING THIS WEEK?
Greatly
Slightly
Not at all
Week Number shown on inhaler label
HAS THE TREAT- MENT HELPED YOU DURING THIS WEEK?
Greatly
Slightly
Not at all

Fig. 6.3

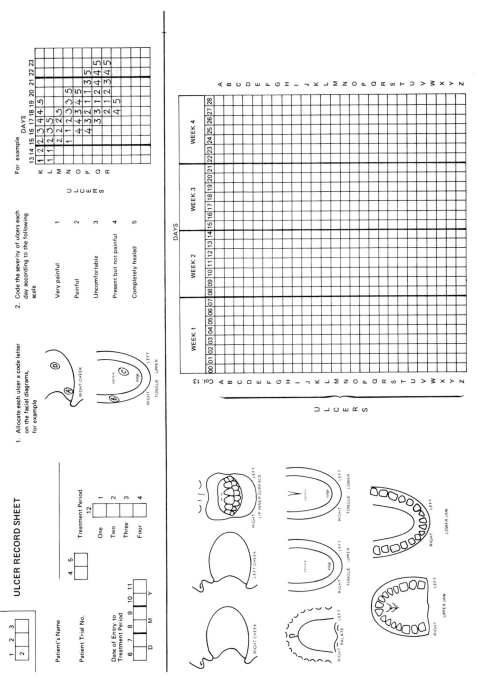

Fig. 6.4

**THE BOLLINGTON STUDY OF HYPERTENSION IN THE ELDERLY**

Patient No. [1 2 3 4]   Record [1][1] (5 6)

Surname _____

Forename _____

Address _____

_____

Occupation _____

Screening Date (9 10 11 12 13 14)

Sex (15)  M [ ] 1   F [ ] 2

Date of Birth (16 17 18 19 20 21)

---

**INITIAL SCREEN**

Systolic B.P. (22 23 24) [ ][ ][ ]

Diastolic B.P. (25 26 27) [ ][ ][ ]

| | Angina | Card. Infarct. | Strokes | Tran.Strokes | Mental. Conf. | Dizzy Spells | Vertigo | Drop. Attacks | Syncopy | Int. Claudtn. | |
|---|---|---|---|---|---|---|---|---|---|---|---|
| | 28 | 29 | 30 | 31 | 32 | 33 | 34 | 35 | 36 | 37 | |
| Normal | | | | | | | | | | | 1 |
| Abnormal | | | | | | | | | | | 2 |

Smoking (38)

| None | 1 |
| <10 | 2 |
| 11–20 | 3 |
| >20 | 4 |
| Pipe | 5 |
| Cigars | 6 |

---

Record (5 6) [1][2]

**INITIAL EXAMINATION**

Date (9 10 11 12 13 14)

Systolic B.P. (16 17 18)

Diastolic B.P. (19 20 21)

Height (22 23) [ ] ins.   Weight (24 25 26) [ ] lbs.   Ht. Rate (27 28 29)

| | Ht. Rhythm | Apex Beat | Syst.Murmers | Dias.Murmers | Basal Creps | Lung Signs | Raised Ven. Pres | Ankle Oedema | Retinoscope Ab. | Femoral Pulses | Abdom. bruit | Abdom.masses | Longtrack signs | Cervical Bruit | Ankle Pulses |
|---|---|---|---|---|---|---|---|---|---|---|---|---|---|---|---|
| | 30 | 31 | 32 | 33 | 34 | 35 | 36 | 37 | 38 | 39 | 40 | 41 | 42 | 43 | 44 |
| Normal | | | | | | | | | | | | | | | |
| Abnormal | | | | | | | | | | | | | | | |

---

**R.C.P.M.S. Questionnaire** (43 44) [ ][ ]

Urine Sugar (45)
Pres. [ ] 1
Abs. [ ] 2

Albumin. (46)
Pres. [ ] 1
Abs. [ ] 2

**E.C.G.** (47 48 49)

Chest X-Ray (56)
Normal [ ] 1
Card Enlgt. [ ] 2
Lung Dis. [ ] 3

**Microscopy** (50)
Normal [ ] 1
Abnormal [ ] 2

Hb (57)
<10 [ ] 1
10–14 [ ] 2
>14 [ ] 3

**Culture** (51)

**Lipo. Profile** (52)
Normal [ ] 1
Type II [ ] 2
Type IV [ ] 3

**Fibrinogen** (53 54 55)

Blood Urea (58 59 60)

Blood Sugar (61 62 63)

S.Uric Acid (64 65)

Na. (66 67 68)

Pot. (69 70)

Cholesterol (71 72 73)

Fig. 6.5

| SURNAME | FORENAMES | No. | | Record |
|---|---|---|---|---|

No. 1 2 3 4   Record 5

[boxes: 1 2 3 4]   [box: 3]

**A**

| | 7 | Date 8 9 10 11 12 13 |
|---|---|---|
| Control | 1 | [boxes] |
| 50 mgm x 2 | 2 | |
| 100 mgm x 2 | 3 | 14 15 16 Systolic B.P. [boxes] |
| 5 mgm Bend | 4 | |
| 10 mgm Bend | 5 | 17 18 19 |
| Therapy discont. | 6 | Diastolic B.P. [boxes] |

Comment

**B**

| | 7 | Date 8 9 10 11 12 13 |
|---|---|---|
| Control | 1 | [boxes] |
| 50 mgm x 2 | 2 | |
| 100 mgm x 2 | 3 | 14 15 16 Systolic B.P. [boxes] |
| 5 mgm Bend | 4 | |
| 10 mgm Bend | 5 | 17 18 19 |
| Therapy discont. | 6 | Diastolic B.P. [boxes] |

Comment

**C**

| | 7 | Date 8 9 10 11 12 13 |
|---|---|---|
| Control | 1 | [boxes] |
| 50 mgm x 2 | 2 | |
| 100 mgm x 2 | 3 | 14 15 16 Systolic B.P. [boxes] |
| 5 mgm Bend | 4 | |
| 10 mgm Bend | 5 | 17 18 19 |
| Therapy discont. | 6 | Diastolic B.P. [boxes] |

Comment

**D**

| | 7 | Date 8 9 10 11 12 13 |
|---|---|---|
| Control | 1 | [boxes] |
| 50 mgm x 2 | 2 | |
| 100 mgm x 2 | 3 | 14 15 16 Systolic B.P. [boxes] |
| 5 mgm Bend | 4 | |
| 10 mgm Bend | 5 | 17 18 19 |
| Therapy discont. | 6 | Diastolic B.P. [boxes] |

Comment

**E**

| | 7 | Date 8 9 10 11 12 13 |
|---|---|---|
| Control | 1 | [boxes] |
| 50 mgm x 2 | 2 | |
| 100 mgm x 2 | 3 | 14 15 16 Systolic B.P. [boxes] |
| 5 mgm Bend | 4 | |
| 10 mgm Bend | 5 | 17 18 19 |
| Therapy discont. | 6 | Diastolic B.P. [boxes] |

Comment

**F**

| | 7 | Date 8 9 10 11 12 13 |
|---|---|---|
| Control | 1 | [boxes] |
| 50 mgm x 2 | 2 | |
| 100 mgm x 2 | 3 | 14 15 16 Systolic B.P. [boxes] |
| 5 mgm Bend | 4 | |
| 10 mgm Bend | 5 | 17 18 19 |
| Therapy discont. | 6 | Diastolic B.P. [boxes] |

Comment

**G**

| | 7 | Date 8 9 10 11 12 13 |
|---|---|---|
| Control | 1 | [boxes] |
| 50 mgm x 2 | 2 | |
| 100 mgm x 2 | 3 | 14 15 16 Systolic B.P. [boxes] |
| 5 mgm Bend | 4 | |
| 10 mgm Bend | 5 | 17 18 19 |
| Therapy discont. | 6 | Diastolic B.P. [boxes] |

Comment

**H**

| | 7 | Date 8 9 10 11 12 13 |
|---|---|---|
| Control | 1 | [boxes] |
| 50 mgm x 2 | 2 | |
| 100 mgm x 2 | 3 | 14 15 16 Systolic B.P. [boxes] |
| 5 mgm Bend | 4 | |
| 10 mgm Bend | 5 | 17 18 19 |
| Therapy discont. | 6 | Diastolic B.P. [boxes] |

Comment

Fig. 6.6

## 'VIVALAN' IN DEPRESSION IN GENERAL PRACTICE

G.P. NAME _____ NO. | 1 | 2 | 3 |

ADDRESS _____

Patients Initials [        ]   No. | 4 | 5 |   Age | 6 | 7 |   Sex   M | | 1 / F | | 2   8

| SYMPTOMS SEVERITY SCORING<br>0 — Absent   3 — Moderate<br>1 — Minimal   4 — Severe<br>2 — Mild   5 — Intolerable | | Col. ENTRY | VISIT No. 1 | VISIT No. 2 | Col. | ENTRY |
|---|---|---|---|---|---|---|
| DEPRESSION | | 9 | | | 29 | Other Drugs |
| ANXIETY | | 10 | | | 30 | |
| INABILITY TO CONCENTRATE | | 11 | | | 31 | Side Effects |
| ALTERED SLEEP PATTERN | | 12 | | | 32 | VISIT 2 |
| FATIGUE/LASSITUDE | | 13 | | | 33 | Other Drugs |
| LOST APPETITE | | 14 | | | 34 | |
| LIBIDO LOSS | | 15 | | | 35 | Side Effects |
| GLOBAL ASSESSMENT | BETTER | 16/1 | | | 36/1 | |
| | SAME | 16/2 | | | 36/2 | |
| | WORSE | 16/3 | | | 36/3 | Trial completed |
| SIDE EFFECTS | PRESENT | 17/1 | | | 37/1 | Patient withdrawn |
| | ABSENT | 17/2 | | | 37/2 | If withdrawn — due to Non-effective |
| OTHER DRUGS | YES | 18/1 | | | 38/1 | Side effects |
| | NO | 18/2 | | | 38/2 | Other Causes |

Under ENTRY column: VISIT 1 — Other Drugs; Side Effects.

39 — Trial completed | 1 ; Patient withdrawn | 2
40 — Non-effective | 1 ; Side effects | 2 ; Other Causes | 3

Comments, including details if withdrawn

Signed..........................................................................Date...................................

Fig. 6.7

**IMPERIAL CHEMICAL INDUSTRIES LTD.**
**PHARMACEUTICALS DIVISION**

**CLINICAL TRIAL OF 'VIVALAN'**
**(VILOXAZINE HYDROCHLORIDE)**
**IN DEPRESSIVE ILLNESS IN GENERAL PRACTICE**

### INTRODUCTION AND AIMS

'Vivalan' is a new antidepressant of novel chemical structure produced by the Pharmaceuticals Division of I.C.I. Limited. It has been shown in controlled clinical trials to be a rapidly acting antidepressant producing little or no sedation and is virtually devoid of anticholinergic properties.

The aim of this study is to assess the value of 'Vivalan' in the treatment of mild to moderate depression in general practice with particular reference to the more common target symptoms.

### PROCEDURE

Five patients with mild to moderate depression who would normally be treated with a tricyclic antidepressant should be chosen for the study. Their agreement to participate should be obtained. Patients under 18 years of age and anyone taking phenytoin (Epanutin) should be excluded. Although animal tests show that 'Vivalan' is not teratogenic, pregnant women should also be excluded.

When first seen, the patient's name or initials, age and sex should be entered overleaf. The overall severity of his symptoms should be scored on a 0 to 5 basis as follows.

| | | |
|---|---|---|
| 0 = absent | 2 = mild | 4 = severe |
| 1 = minimal | 3 = moderate | 5 = intolerable |

Patients are then given 'Vivalan' at a dose of 1 x 50 mg tablet three times a day, tablets to be taken with meals. Patients are reviewed at weekly intervals for two weeks. Each time the patient is reviewed, the score of depression, anxiety and other target symptoms should be recorded. A global assessment should be done and the presence and nature of possible side effects recorded. If the patient is withdrawn from the study, the reason should be noted in the space provided. Details of other drugs given should be recorded. The trial will last for two weeks.

All patient data should be recorded on the record sheet overleaf. The ICI medical representative will collect the completed record sheets from you as soon as these become available and also will make available further supplies of tablets or record sheets and will give any assistance in filling in the record sheet which may be required.

Fig. 6.8

We appreciate that no matter how many questions appear on a record form and no matter how many sections there are to complete, it will still be necessary to permit the clinician to add extra data and information. The record form cannot cope with every possible situation in the clinical interview. In an attempt to overcome this problem we include in the form an area where the clinician can write any additional information and ask the question 'Comments', Yes/No. When this is completed it allows us to find within the system the patient visit numbers of all the records which have additional information. These records are then examined visually using a microfilm reader.

Side effects present a problem to which, as yet, we have found no definite solution. We prefer to include in the record an item by item list of side effects and for the physician to ask the patients about each item. Our transatlantic colleagues refer to this as 'laundry listing' and state that it plants ideas in the patients' minds. We insist that our approach acts as an *aide memoire* and that the open-ended questions: 'How are you feeling today?' or 'Have you noticed any ill effects from the treatment?' do not indicate to the patient that he should then discuss his vivid dreams, his constipation or his loss of libido. Absence of any reference to these side effects in the record would indicate that since they were not recorded, they were not present. It could just as easily be that they were not considered at interview. The answer to the problem of side effects probably lies somewhere between the two approaches. Our recent clinical trial record forms have included sections for both volunteered and elicited answers.

The third common problem in form design is the use of the comparative question and answer, 'How is your angina?' - Better/Same/Worse. Answers to these questions create the further questions: 'Better than what and when?' This is usually answered by 'better than it was last time'. Examination of the records reveals that 'last time' it was coded as 'same'. Linkage of these comparative answers over a series of visits usually reveals that every individual in the trial has a unique response pattern.

When a trial has finally been completed, all the time, money and effort have been expended and patients return to open therapy, the only item remaining is the record. If it has been well designed and completed, it holds the total data representing all the work. It does not matter where the data arose, from operating theatre to general practice, in the United Kingdom or abroad; it does not matter what it is about, from surgery to psychiatry, from teeth to toes; it does not matter how you are going to handle the data, from simple manual systems to IBM or ICL computers; a well designed record form presents the information in a manner compatible to all systems.

Clinical trials are an expensive, time consuming, but essential aspect of the pharmaceutical industry. This outlay is best underwritten by the most careful acquisition of clinical trial data. At ICI Pharmaceuticals Division, we spend a considerable time on form design, to ensure that we have a correct, accurate, complete, uniform data record. It is only from such records that valid evaluations can be made.

REFERENCES

Blackeney-Edwards, N.J., Eddins, R.A. & Rhodes, J.J. (1970) Report on the feasibility of a clinical trials package. Private communication.

McLean, E.R., Foote, S.V. & Wagner, G. (1975) The collection and processing of medical history data. *Meth. Inf. Med.* 14, 150 - 163.

Mellner, C., Selander, H. & Wolodarski, J. (1976) The computerised problem orientated medical record at Karolinska Hospital - format and function, users' acceptance and patient attitude to questionnaire. *Meth. Inf. Med.* 15, 11 - 20.

# 7.   The Choice of Investigator

E. S. SNELL

Meeting the objectives of investigations with drugs, and the speed with which this is done, are influenced in a major way by the independent doctors undertaking the work. Hence it is worth spending time and trouble to choose investigators with care. The nature of the proposed study, will largely decide the professional and scientific qualifications and the patients and facilities required from the investigator. Personal attributes are most important requirements for workers in drug trials. These may be decisive in choosing the particular doctor from a number similarly qualified scientifically. In many ways they are the most important. Departure from the ideal in other respects can often be made good, but nothing can make up for serious deficiencies in personal qualities. This chapter is intended to apply to investigations within the UK, but much would also be appropriate to foreign studies; into which, unfortunately, British pharmaceutical research is bring increasingly driven.

## Types of studies

Some general points may be made on the type of study. Classification of studies into phases 1, 2, 3 and 4 has no advantage in the UK and merely obscures some definitions. Human research can be divided into: Work done in normal volunteers * before submission to the registration authorities; and clinical studies in patients after approval of such submissions and undertaken either before or after marketing. Additionally the nature of the study is best described by accepted scientific terms as follows:

### Clinical pharmacology

These studies will be suitable for academic research units and teaching hospital centres or will be undertaken in the company itself. It is both acceptable and desirable that most early studies on non-patient volunteers are conducted within the companies' own laboratories, provided that the necessary expertise and facilities are available to ensure safety of the subjects and to make the required observations. Drugs with profound activity may be an exception but many of these would not be tested in normal volunteers at all. Studies outside the company on drug metabolism and kinetics in non-patient volunteers or in patients must be undertaken by those experienced in the methods and with the facilities required for monitoring and safety. The company may

---

*These subjects must be free from known pathology related to likely actions of the drug and not patients under medical surveillance for any other condition. They can best be described as non-patient volunteers.

have to provide special formulations and radioactive labelled drugs as well as methods of drug estimation or themselves undertaken these or other investigations.

Pharmacodynamic studies must also be done by those with the relevant skills, as for example in cardiovascular, respiratory or other organ function tests. It is one thing to make elaborate measurements of physiological functions with complicated techniques, and yet another to ensure that it is done so that the results are susceptible to valid interpretation.

Information on human toxicology is usually obtained by careful clinical observation and standard tests of body function as a by-product of studies with other objectives. If specialised clinical observations are needed, such as assessment of the psychic response, or special investigations such as tissue biopsy, genetic or immunological studies, the investigator must have the appropriate knowledge and facilities.

*Early clinical studies*

These should be undertaken in hospitals with suitable patients; teaching centres are especially suitable. The doctors' speciality will correspond with the likely clinical use of the drug so that, for example, dermatologists will be chosen for dermatological drugs and anaesthetists for anaesthetics. However, the type of speciality may not be mandatory for a drug with a wider use, such as an antibiotic, and other factors may commend a particular investigator. In this event the type of investigation can be tailored to the clinical interests and work of the investigator. The art of clinical trials is to plan a series of investigations so that, as a whole, they provide the broad body of information required but so that each one best fits the interests and patients of the individual investigator. The information usually sought in these early studies is essentially clinical. There should be careful observation of the disease process (monitored as far as possible by relevant tests) in response to open use of the drug perhaps at various doses. Those skilled already in this art, especially with new drugs, will form the most valuable investigators. Some clinicians feel that they are unable adequately to assess the response of disease to a drug without a control group of patients treated with a standard remedy. Such clinicians will be helpful only in later stages of the clinical work.

*Later clinical studies*

The studies will usually be controlled comparisons with other drugs, probably by double-blind administration. More than careful clinical observation is here required from the investigator. Scrupulous attention to the details of a complicated protocol will be needed, probably in large numbers of patients. Experience is valuable but not essential. There is nothing inherently difficult, or specialised, about carrying out a planned trial providing the doctor has the medical skills and personal qualities needed and will devote sufficient time and trouble. Detailed action may be left to a junior member of medical staff, or ancillary. These studies will be well suited both to non-teaching and teaching hospitals.

*Post marketing studies*

When a drug has been marketed there will probably be publications on it or it will be well known to experts in the field so that there may be little to do of interest to academic research units or teaching hospitals but other appropriate hospital doctors may be willing to continue the work. General practice studies can now also be considered.

## Types of clinical centres

It is worth considering in more detail some of the general advantages and disadvantages for drug research in the different types of centres available for cooperation.

### Research and academic units

These contain the highest levels of knowledge, intelligence and facilities for their special subject. They may also contain an attractive concentration of well documented patients. However, their interests will be only in prestigious work of high scientific content. Recent debate on pure and applied research has improved the prospects for the type of well defined applied research needed by industry, providing the study has the required degree of innate scientific interest. Other advantages can result from collaboration with such units. They can provide expert and independent helpful criticisms of other data from the company's own research or from elsewhere. They can also suggest useful ideas and new methodology for future studies or even modification of the product.

Departments of clinical pharmacology can offer particular benefits in these ways. The special interest of the 17 Chairs now devoted to this subject should be well known to all those responsible for drug studies. Sometimes these units expect rather large grants, especially for a less exciting research proposal. This must be allowed for in the drug development budget if this type of high quality work is required.

### Other departments in teaching hospitals

Such centres have many of the characteristics of academic units but usually have a closer affinity to practical clinical medicine. However, they carry a heavier load of routine clinical work, less equipment and a smaller staff. Their main requirement for any work that is not already part of their programme is for extra pairs of hands and more facilities. The company can provide these by grants or help from company staff (medical and non-medical) or from the company's laboratory services.

Specialised groups of patients collected as in-patients or out-patients, as in venereal disease, allergy and hypertension, form a valuable source of material for study in both teaching and non-teaching hospitals. A hospital may be entirely devoted to one subject as in psychiatric and submentality hospitals.

### Non-teaching hospitals

In these centres the facilities and time available for research are further curtailed but the enthusiasm for simpler clinical trials may be proportionally increased; such work may be the only type of research feasible. The study must be suitably adapted for the time available for its conduct and not too demanding of special investigations. There is usually the advantage of an abundance of patients in such centres. Staff may need guidance in forming protocols and in arranging the logistics of both drug and patients. Comparatively modest grants, or other provisions, usually provide strong extra motivation. Consultants trained in this way can form valuable allies for further similar studies. Among the benefits to them is the raising of the quality of junior hospital doctors applying for their posts when it is seen that research and publications are possible from them.

For both teaching and non-teaching hospitals the appointment of a 'Research Registrar' funded (partly or wholly) by one or more companies jointly can lead to an ideal situation. The doctor may undertake more than one study at a time under supervision of an experienced hospital consultant and the company. This experience may lead an interested doctor to pursue a specialty in clinical pharmacology or to join a pharmaceutical company. It will be of permanent value to him as an exercise whatever his later career.

Another satisfactory arrangement which offers economy to the company, as well as extra personnel and interesting work to the hospital, is provision of extra part-time medical staff; say to an out-patient clinic undertaking a drug study. Busy full time staff are spared the anguish and overtime of making detailed observations on patients beyond the needs of routine medicine. The trial gets full attention from the part-time extra doctor. For a general practitioner, one or two such out-patient sessions can form an interesting variation in his work. Alternatively, a doctor seeking part-time work, such as a mother, can be a suitable candidate.

It is not always extra doctors that are needed for a study, for extra part time nurses or other ancillary staff can be valuable. For example, nurses (health visitors) can visit homes to follow up clinical responses or collect special investigations of out-patients treated, for instance, with vaccines. Dieticians can supply essential data on nutritional studies by calculating inventories of diets. Technicians may be able to collect blood or other samples from patients at defined times when doctors might not be free to do so.

### Community health and other special centres

Some products, such as vaccines and infant foods, must be tested on subjects who are not hospital patients. For these, cooperation must be sought from appropriate units. They may be clinics for infant welfare or for school children or industrial health centres. The protocol will need to be simple and special investigations minimal, bearing in mind that the time available from the subjects and the investigators is limited. Help for the study as previously outlined will be invaluable for such centres.

### General practice

Some illnesses, such as minor haemorrhoids or less severe degrees of bronchitis and neuroses, are only found in general practice and must be studied there. Also, drug efficacy in some chronic diseases may differ in the domiciliary environment of general practice from that in hospital. Virtually the sole source of untreated patients, if these are required for study, is in general practice. General Practitioners (GP's) with a hospital clinical assistantship in a specialty, such as dermatology, are particularly suitable for research and may do some of the work in that clinic. The obvious disadvantages of such work are the time constraints on the practitioner and the limits of his facilities for investigations. The design of the study must be such that patients can be adequately characterised at entry and on follow up, especially for multicentre trials. If this is done, much useful data can be derived from general practice and the practitioner's work much enriched.

In the long term it is more satisfactory to build one's own panel of GP investigators, paying particular attention to personal qualities, rather than to employ one of the 'professional' readymade groups. Frequent visits to the doctors are advisable to collect data and follow progress. This may be done by either medical or non-medical scientific staff from the medical department but not by sales department staff. Occasional group meetings of all the panel to discuss results is stimulating for them. For diseases easily followed objectively, such as hypertension, a drug study in hospital out-patients can be extended into a few general practices to increase the supply of patients and to offer greater convenience to them.

Unfortunately many so-called GP trials have been disguised marketing exercises rather than true scientific enquiries. This has aroused the suspicions of GPs approached to do *bona fide* studies as well as those reading the published results. It is to be hoped that the reputation of GP trials can be enhanced by more high quality work and that this very valuable potential for research can be better exploited. GP medical centres should have many advantages for this type of work.

Adequate surveillance for the nature and incidence of side effects of marketed drugs is perhaps one of the greatest deficiencies in therapeutics today. Observations in general practice could do much to meet this need if properly organised, perhaps around special hospital centres given the same task or in academic GP units.

## Personal qualities of the investigator

There are many starting points to the choice of a particular investigator. He may be well known by publications and repute for previous work either with the same type of drug or in a special field of medicine, or he may have worked with the company previously on drug trials. Occasionally he may approach the company to undertake studies and this forms a particularly favourable prognostic sign. He may be known socially or professionally. All of these diverse origins may be a useful start to a relationship. Having satisfied scientific and professional requirements one must look closely to personal factors. The personal nature of the clinical investigator especially in relation to the company investigator's own personality should be explored for the two will work closely together: A productive relationhip is more likely when it is a harmonious one. This mutual personal relationship is the key to successful trials and may lead one to work repeatedly on trials with the same investigator.

### Integrity

This quality is doubly important as it affects the interests of the patients, the over-riding consideration in drug trials, as well as the reliability of the results. However carefully a protocol is drawn up to ensure high ethical standards, it is up to the doctor caring for the patients to see that their participation is not detrimental to them. Standards of ethics in the UK are very high. They are supported by various guidelines, such as the Declaration of Helsinki, and practical constraints like hospital ethics committees. It is rare to rule out a potential investigator because his excessive zeal for data might risk the safety of patients. Fortunately it is also rare for fictitious data to be returned by our profession; but it has happened and one hears of checks being undertaken on drug trial results in other countries. A different aspect of the investigator's integrity is his attitude to the company, particularly once the grant has been paid or promised, which can affect the quality and quantity of data as well as any subsequent publications. Mutually agreed studies have been published with only partial, if any, information on the results or their interpretation being sent to the company. If this happens the account of the trial can give an incomplete or even unfair reflection of the drug. One also relies on the doctor's integrity for maintaining confidentiality of the work.

*Motivation*

Many, and different, motives may form an acceptable basis for a doctor's cooperation in a study, but behind most of these one seeks a genuine interest in acquiring new information. A desire for publications, in the interests of personal career progression or advancement of the reputation of a department, forms a common and useful motive.

Particularly in these days of limited financial resources for research, another legitimate motive can be supplied by the prospect of a grant, either to aid the study or to further the professional education of the investigator. However, large personal fees do not form a satisfactory basis for a relationship. The prognosis for trials is good with those consultants who feel that an environment of research is essential training for their undergraduates and postgraduate staff. As a corollary, the outlook for trials is gloomy where the chief feels that all research on patients is an intrusion into good clinical practice.

An excess of enthusiasm from a potential investigator with a profusion of ideas and projects should be received with much caution. Such exaggerated interests are liable to prove vapid and worthwhile data not forthcoming.

*Reliability*

A reliable outcome of the trial rests on a combination of qualities. These include conscientiousness, determination, enthusiasm, leadership (of nursing staff as well as of other doctors), ability to cooperate with others involved in the research (especially with the company), commonsense to pursue the right course in spite of the inevitable difficulties that will arise and, perhaps above all, orderliness: The methodical acquisition and recording of data is unlikely to be achieved except by tidy habits.

In conclusion I emphasize the need to establish a close personal relationship with the investigator based on mutual compatibility, trust and respect. This, together with the right blend of personal qualities and professional skill from the investigator will provide the best assurance of successful clinical trials.

# 8.  Budgeting for Clinical Trials

P. A. NICHOLSON

In the United Kingdom clinical research (a term used in this book only in the context of drug evaluation) is usually carried out in University Departments, in National Health Service Hospitals, or in General Practice.

The objectives of such clinical research are to identify the absolute and comparative pharmacological, therapeutic and toxicological profiles of a drug, thereby enabling it to be registered for sale, or to provide material which, when published, will support its sale by permitting it to be used wisely in an informed way.

Budgeting for clinical trials involves estimating the total expenditure which will be incurred in their 'conception', 'gestation', 'parturition' and subsequent development, including their analysis, reporting and publication.

These costs may be substantial, and may exceed greatly the arbitrary sums which, if asked, we might attribute to them without a detailed examination of all the charges involved. The payments which may be made to a third party to conduct the study may be only a small part of the total resources employed in the trial.

Many studies are conceived. Unfortunately not all of them reach a satisfactory outcome. The cost of the failures should be regarded as an additional overhead on the cost of the successes. This is true for all research activities in the pharmaceutical industry. A clinical trial is not a trivial matter. It represents a substantial investment, which a detailed examination of the costs will confirm. The costs will be examined in this chapter and presented as a basis for company budgeting. In this context they can be divided into two main groups:

1. Internal costs
2. External costs

## Internal costs

These include a proportion of the salaries of all those in the company involved in the planning, co-ordination and supervision of a study and the analysis and presentation of the results. A trial is essentially a team effort and the more sophisticated the company, the larger the team will be. The members of the team and their main responsibilities may resemble the following:

| *Personnel* | *Function* |
| --- | --- |
| Medical Adviser | Overall supervision of the study. Designing the protocol. Assisting in the analysis of data. Writing the paper (jointly). |

| | |
|---|---|
| Clinical Research Associate | Regular monitoring of progress. Checking the adequacy of data input. Checking supplies, packaging and labelling in the pharmacy. |
| Secretary | Arranging appointments for principals. Travel arrangements. Preparing protocols and record cards. All correspondence and filing. |
| Statistician | Designing the protocol, record cards, randomisation and code break. Analysing and reporting on the data. |
| Pharmacist | Production of materials in appropriate registrable forms for use in the project. |
| Packer | Packaging and labelling of supplies. Despatch of trial materials. |

The cost of this team is clearly substantial. But in addition to the proportion of the salaries allocated to any one study, a proportion of the overheads should also be allocated. 'Overheads' include power, rent, heating, rates, staff canteen, pensions, other insurances, depreciation, interest etc.

Internal costs also include the cost of materials, such as the following:

*Packaging materials .* Bottles. Stoppers. Dessicants. Cotton wool. Cardboard cartons. Wrappings.

*Printing materials.* Record cards. Protocols. Labels for bottles.

*Raw materials.* Drugs.

In addition, some internal services may be itemised separately. For example, few medical departments enjoy their own computing facility, but most have access to a computer within their company. This is usually a central service and charged to a department according to usage. Special literature surveys may be done prior to embarking on a clinical trial. These too must be costed.

An example is given in Table 8.1, based upon a team such as has been described. Several assumptions have been made. A medical adviser may be concerned with clinical trials for approximately 60 per cent of his time. He could supervise about 15 clinical research projects actively. Four per cent of his salary and overheads, therefore, should be allocated to any single study. A Clinical Research Associate (C.R.A.), usually a non medically qualified science graduate, will spend all of his time on clinical trials. He may be involved in twice as many projects as the adviser but in a less profound manner - perhaps these number 30 in total. Any single study will 'cost' 3.3 per cent of his salary and overheads. The commitment of other personnel to a single study can be estimated in a similar way. In Table 8.1 an outline of the order of the financial commitment for personnel is given.

Material costs vary according to the dimensions of the study, the sophistication of the record cards, the nature of the drugs involved and the duration of treatment, but can cost several hundred pounds. Computing charges vary according to the nature of

Table 8.1  Estimation of internal costs per trial per annum

| Person | Salary £ p.a. | Overheads £(Salary÷2) | Involvement % | Cost £ |
|---|---|---|---|---|
| Medical Adviser | 8500 | 4250 | 4.0 | 510 |
| C.R.A. | 4500 | 2250 | 3.3 | 227.75 |
| Secretary | 2500 | 1250 | 2.0 | 75 |
| Statistician | 4000 | 2000 | 2.0 | 120 |
| Pharmacist | 6750 | 3375 | 0.5 | 50.63 |
| Packer | 2500 | 1250 | 0.5 | 18.73 |
| Material costs | | | | 350 |
| Computing charges | | | | 200 |
| | | | Total | 1552.13 |

the demands and the time involved.

In short, internal costs will probably exceed £1500 per average trial, but can vary substantially up to several thousands of pounds in complex multicentre studies.

## External costs

Many of these costs are beyond one's own control and this introduces an area of uncertainty in budgetary planning. However, the costs can be categorised along the following lines.

*Cost of services.*  Travel, hospitality and accommodation of company personnel or third parties.

Postage, telephone and telex charges.

Delivery charges (if not postal) for goods.

Dispensing fee to pharmacist (if materials are supplied in bulk and require special packaging).

Travel and accommodation charges are the largest feature in the service costs. Clearly it is more expensive for London based companies to maintain a personal contact with trialists in Aberdeen, Edinburgh, Glasgow and Belfast than in Middlesex.

## *Payments to clinicians*

It is necessary here to emphasise that the success of studies depends upon the motivation and involvement of all the people involved. Just as the medical department within a company plans a trial on a team basis, so also is the trial usually conducted on a team basis. The contributions of all the members of a team should be recognised. Doctors participating in trials may be assuming an increased work load and increased responsibility. Moreover, they are providing a specialist professional service for which their experience and training particularly qualifies them. This should be recognised and rewarded. If they are inconvenienced by additional work, or if by participating in the study they are thereby unable to maintain their income in more regular ways, they should be adequately compensated. The level of payment should be related to the amount of work carried out.

The Medicopharmaceutical Forum (1974) suggested that payments to clinicians should be approved by the ethics committee or its equivalent which approves the trial protocol. The Forum also specifically mentioned the risk that such financial recognition could adversely affect the normal doctor patient relationship. In my experience, this is a remote hazard.

All agreements regarding financial support of any kind must be reached before starting the study and should be written agreements.

Upon what are such agreements with clinicians based? One practice is to estimate the likely time per week during which the clinician will be involved in the study. If this is the equivalent of one half day, then it would be regarded as the equivalent of one session, and so on. The reward for one session can be worked out from the salary scales printed in the British Medical Journal. At present they are shown in Table 8.2.

Table 8.2  Full time N.H.S. (hospital) salaries

|                            | £ p.a.           |
| -------------------------- | ---------------- |
| House Officer              | 2859 - 3294      |
| Senior House Officer       | 3663 - 4152      |
| Registrar                  | 4152 - 5109      |
| Senior Registrar           | 4818 - 6279      |
| Part Time Medical Officer  | 610 *            |
| Hospital Practitioner Grade| 610 -   826 *    |
| Medical Assistant          | 4548 - 7812      |
| Consultant                 | 7536 - 10,689    |

* Half day per week per year.

If it is possible to employ a general practitioner one session a week to perform a specific duty for a specific reward, this is often more satisfactory than recognising that a registrar already employed is doing the work, and then making an equivalent financial contribution to a department's general funds. Establishing a direct relationship between the appointment, the task and the reward can be very important to the success of the study.

An alternative method of reimbursing clinicians is to pay a fee for each item of service. One example is to pay a fee for each adequately completed record card. 'Adequate' means that it can usefully contribute to the analysis.

However, if a clinician is being reimbursed on a sessional basis, or an item of service basis, it is probably wise to recognise the cooperation of the unit by making an additional *ex gratia* contribution to its funds.

*Payments to other staff*

The National Economic Development Office report (1972) rightly emphasised that there were two particular areas where real difficulties were encountered in clinical trials: Firstly in the administration of the drugs: Secondly in the collection of the appropriate samples at the right time and in the correct manner. A third difficulty was mentioned also, the incomplete assembly of data which leads to incomplete results. It cannot be emphasised too much that nursing and technical staff involved in a trial should enjoy proper recognition of their expertise and additional reward for duties undertaken in excess of normal. Financial arrangements can also be reached on a sessional or item of service basis here too. For example, technicians' salaries are published by the Professional and Technical 'B' Whitely Council.

An example of external staffing costs is shown in Table 8.3. In the area of technical assistance, it should be clear that the obligation to reimburse is limited to those investigations performed in excess of normal medical care. If these investigations are itemised and costed individually, a wise medical adviser will obtain quotations from commercial laboratories performing the same service to see whether he can negotiate more acceptable terms outside the hospital or university. Several commercial concerns provide such laboratory services. However, the convenience of a service on the spot is considerable and may outweigh economic considerations.

Table 8.3   External costs per annum

| Staff | Commitment | Cost £ |
|---|---|---|
| Hospital Practitioner | 1 Session/week | 826 |
| Technician | 1 Session/week | 340 |
| Hospital Sister | 1 Session/week | 275 |
| | Total | 1,441 |

In some departments, it is preferred that all monies are donated to research funds or travel accounts. Nevertheless, a reasonable fee for the total service can be estimated on the above basis.

### Payments to volunteers

The W.H.O. (1968) recognises that volunteers in some clinical trials will be financially rewarded for their participation. Sometimes the reward is to encourage participation. Sometimes it is incidental to participation. However, the reward should never be sufficient to encourage submission to unreasonably hazardous procedures, which may now be prevented by the widespread existence of ethics committees. There are, unfortunately, no 'hard and fast' rules for the size of such payments.

### Payments to patients

Out of pocket expenses should be reimbursed; that is, loss of earnings and fares in attending for additional consultations. But there must be no inducement to participate.

### Miscellaneous costs

Indemnity insurance premiums and any publication charges merit consideration. The company may be called upon to provide the former. The company may have to consider the second for several reasons. It may wish to control the timing of the publication, and may wish to ensure that the report is published simultaneously with others on the same topic. It may wish to provide simultaneously issues in alternative languages, facilities which are easier to come by in some journals than others.

The costs of studies include internal costs and external costs. In each example the charges quoted are per annum. The average clinical trial usually takes more than a year. The external charges quoted only reimburse the costs of the study but do not add a monetary incentive to a department to conduct the trial. This may require an additional payment.

Finally, establishing clinical research activities is a business. It is our duty to ensure that resources are used economically. When compounds are inherently exciting, there is rarely any need to use financial stimuli to establish their evaluation. When they are inherently dull, financial benefit is needed as a motive.

## REFERENCES

Medicopharmaceutical Forum (1974) A report by the Forum's working party on clinical trials. *Medicopharmaceutical Forum,* 19.

National Economic Development Office (1972) Focus on pharmaceuticals. *A Report by the Pharmaceuticals Working Party of the Chemicals E.D.C.* London: Her Majesty's Stationery Office.

W.H.O. Scientific Group Report (1968) Principles for the clinical evaluation of drugs. *W.H.O. Technical Report Series,* **403**, 19.

# 9. Statistical Aspects of Trial Design

K. D. MACRAE

A clinical trial is a scientific experiment applied to the solution of clinical problems. To emphasise the scientific nature of such studies, they are often referred to as prospective, randomised, controlled clinical trials, and this description is sometimes further amplified by the terms 'single blind' or 'double blind'. The increasing acceptance by the medical profession of the clinical trial as the best, perhaps only, means for obtaining sound information about the value of alternative treatments has been referred to as a major advance in medicine (Fisher, 1973). However, as Fisher points out, labelling a study as 'prospective', 'randomised', 'controlled', or indeed anything else, does not ensure the worth of the data produced.

In common with all scientific experiments, clinical trials are designed with the aim of eliminating all sources of systematic bias affecting the resulting measurements, except the effect of the treatment difference being investigated. This means that the experimental design must adequately control possible sources of unwanted bias, and that the measurements on the patients must be unaffected by the experimenter's opinions about the relative effectiveness of the treatments being compared. First, then, a brief word about the measurement problem.

## Measurement in clinical trials

A measurement made on a patient in a clinical trial must fulfill certain criteria if the trial is to produce satisfactory answers.

First, and most important, the measurement must be RELEVANT to the clinical problem being investigated. Very often, several measures of treatment success or failure are relevant, and it is most important that undesirable effects of treatment are considered along with the hoped for therapeutic effect.

Secondly, the measurement should be free from OBSERVER BIAS, and this can be achieved in either of two ways. Objective measures, such as survival time, weight, or the results of haematological or biochemical investigations, are largely immune from possible observer bias. However, much that is important in medicine depends on a subjective evaluation by the doctor or the patient. For this reason so called 'blind' trials are very desirable, in which either the assessing doctor, or the patient (single blind trials) or both (double blind trials) are unaware of the treatment the patient has received.

Thirdly, the measurement should be ACCURATE, in the sense that the level of accuracy is appropriate to the clinical situation being studied. For example, it is difficult to imagine a trial in which survival time would have to be measured to the nearest minute, or even to the nearest hour, although this might be technically feasible.

On the other hand, it can be very difficult to obtain a sufficient degree of accuracy for certain measurements. In a trial comparing analgesics, it will be necessary to find the degree of pain relief achieved by each of two preparations, either by comparing two groups of patients each having been treated with one of the analgesics, or by administering both drugs to the same group of patients on two separate occasions. In either case it would be necessary to measure pain in some way with a degree of accuracy that is capable of showing any differences between the two preparations. In many clinical trials the clinician will have to make subjective assessments of the degree of improvement in observable lesions, or of the results of radiological or isotope scanning investigations. This problem requires particular attention during the design of the data report form, and one of the major tasks in drawing up a trial protocol can be the precise definition of the grades of success the treatments can achieve.

### Experimental design

The primary aim of the design of any experiment, including a clinical trial, is to ensure the absence of CONFOUNDING, that is to avoid any systematic differences between the treatments being compared other than those deliberately introduced by the experimenter. The fundamental way in which possible confounding is avoided is by randomisation, usually by randomly allocating patients into one of the possible treatment groups or, where the patients are to receive both of two treatments, by randomly deciding for each patient which of the two treatments is to be received first. This ensures that confounding resulting from selection bias is avoided.

Sometimes, however, trials are seen in which confounding has been introduced by the experimenter, and the danger here is that this may be ignored in interpreting the results of the trial. A field of study in which treatment confounding is quite common is primary treatment for operable breast cancer. It is not unusual to see a trial comparing a less radical operation plus a high dose of radiotherapy with more radical surgery plus a lower dose of radiation, or perhaps no radiation at all. In such instances, it must be remembered that the trial is not just comparing the two operations, but two complete treatment regimens, the effect of surgery being confounded with the effect of radiotherapy. In a nutshell, absence of confounding means that there is only one systematic difference between the two situations being compared, and that difference is the one being studied by the investigator.

A further aim of an experimental design is to use the subject or patient resources efficiently. The simplest situation, the comparison of two treatments, will be discussed, although the principles can be generalised to the comparison of three or more treatments. This problem is usually one of deciding whether to use two separate groups of patients, one for each treatment, or whether to use paired observations, either by arranging the patients into pairs having similar and supposedly relevant characteristics, (for example, age, sex, duration or severity of illness) or by applying both treatments to each patient. Randomisation is an essential part of all these possible procedures. When the treatments are compared using two independent groups of subjects, the patients are allocated to one or other treatment group randomly, once it has been decided that they are suitable for the trial. When paired observations are to be used, with one member of each pair receiving one treatment and the other member the other treatment, the choice of treatment within each pair is made randomly. If each patient is to receive both treatments, the order of administration is decided on randomly. In the usual terminology of experimental design, the use of two independent groups is referred to as a completely randomised design, and the use of paired measurements is the randomised block design, where the patients or patient pairs are blocks and the choice of treatment within a block is randomised.

How is the choice between the unpaired and paired designs made? The aim of the paired design is to reduce the effect of individual differences between patients, and this is most effective when the same patients receive each treatment. A further benefit is that the number of patients required for a given amount of data is halved (in the two-treatment situation) when patients receive both treatments. Finally, the paired design is the most effective way of assessing a change such as the effect of a weight loss programme, when the paired observations are the weights of the subjects before and after the programme. However, it may be either impossible or misleading to apply both treatments to each patient. The impossibility of performing both of two types of gastric surgery, or of using each of two antibiotics to cure the same infection, is clear. More dangerous, however, is the possibility of 'carry over effects', in which the patient is changed by the first treatment in some subtle way. For this reason, the crossover design has been used, in which possible carryover effects can be partially checked (MacRae, 1969). With matched pairs of patients, the practical difficulty of matching can be a problem, especially if many unmatched cases are left at the end of the trial. The effectiveness of the matching depends on knowledge of the relevant matching variables. For these reasons, it is often necessary or advisable to use the completely randomised (unpaired) design.

### Size of the study

Often, the first question with which the potential clinical trialist approaches his statistical adviser is 'how many patients do I need in order to find out if treatment A is better than treatment B?' For reasons of economy, and because the answer will be available sooner, it is desirable to use as few cases as possible in a clinical trial. It is also ethically desirable to use the smallest number of patients possible. If one of the treatments is superior, patients are not treated unnecessarily using the inferior treatment because the trial has continued too long. On the other hand it is a waste of time and effort to carry out a clinical trial with so few patients that no definite conclusions can be drawn. Again, there is an ethical consideration. The patients in such a trial will have received a treatment of doubtful efficacy, and possibly have been subjected to uncomfortable investigations, without the primary research aim being achieved. Their cooperation, and any inconvenience, will have been in vain, not because a superior treatment did not exist, but because the trial was too small.

The size of a trial depends on three factors, namely, the desired precision or sensitivity of the trial, and the probabilities of each of the two sorts of statistical error. The precision of the trial affects the number of patients required. The more exact the answer being sought, the greater will be the necessary number of patients. Similarly, to make both sorts of statistical error less likely, more patients are needed.

The meaning of trial precision or sensitivity can be illustrated by some hypothetical examples. Suppose that the best established treatment for a disease achieves a

75 per cent 'cure' rate, and that a trial is being planned to see if a new treatment can improve on this figure. The clinical trialist must then decide how small a treatment difference he wishes to detect. Is it worthwhile finding a new treatment that improves the cure rate by 5 per cent, or would an improvement of at least 10 per cent or even more be necessary for the new treatment to be a worthwhile advance? It must be emphasised that this is a value judgement which the statistician is certainly not qualified to make. For quantitative measurements, such as weight and blood pressure, the precision of the trial is expressed as the number of standard deviations the trial is intended to detect. Kastenbaum, Hoel and Bowman (1970) give a hypothetical example where the mean life span of a strain of mice was estimated to be 125 weeks, with a standard deviation of 20 weeks: An experiment is being considered in which the reduction in life span caused by X-radiation is to be studied. If, on average, a five week reduction in life span is of interest, the experiment must be capable of detecting 5/20 or 0.25 standard deviations of a difference. These examples will be used to illustrate the choice of a suitable sample size.

As was said earlier, the two sorts of statistical error also determine the size of the investigation. The TYPE I ERROR can be defined as claiming that the two treatments differ, when in fact they do not. The TYPE II ERROR is when the two treatments do actually differ, but the trial fails to demonstrate this difference. Both sorts of error are highly undesirable. Clinical trials, and indeed all experiments, deal with samples of data. This means that the results are susceptible to sampling error, and that the correct conclusions may not be reached. It is important to keep the probabilities of the two sorts of error very small. The maximum acceptable probability of either sort of error is usually set at P = 0.05 (or 5 per cent). Thus, a 5 per cent SIGNIFI-CANCE LEVEL for a clinical trial means that the maximum acceptable probability of a Type I Error has been set at 5 per cent. The probability of making a Type II Error is often stated by expressing the converse, the probability of NOT making a Type II Error. This will be 95 per cent if the maximum acceptable error probability is 5 per cent. The probability of not making a Type II Error is sometimes termed the POWER of the experiment, and this is the probability that the study will find a treatment difference, if in fact there is one.

We are now in a position to consider the numbers that would be required in the hypothetical studies mentioned earlier. In the example where the accepted treatment achieved a 75 per cent cure rate, table 9.1 can be used to determine the number of

Table 9.1 Numbers of subjects per group required to detect the difference between two percentages, for significance level = 5 per cent and power = 95 per cent (modified from Cochran and Cox, 1957)

| Initial Percentage | Improvement to be detected | | | | |
| | 5% | 10% | 15% | 25% | 50% |
| --- | --- | --- | --- | --- | --- |
| 5% | 701 | 220 | 115 | 52 | 19 |
| 10% | 1128 | 324 | 160 | 67 | 21 |
| 25% | 2075 | 542 | 251 | 95 | 24 |
| 50% | 2589 | 641 | 280 | 95 | -- |
| 75% | 1806 | 410 | 160 | -- | -- |
| 90% | 701 | -- | -- | -- | -- |

cases required. It can be seen that 1806 patients per group, meaning 3612 in all (two groups) would be required to detect a 5 per cent improvement, at the stated Type I and II Error rates. A 10 per cent improvement could be detected with 410 per group, 820 in all, and a 15 per cent improvement with 160 per group, a total of 320 patients. In the example mentioned from Kastenbaum et al (1970) the treatment difference (T) was 0.25 standard deviations. This can be seen from table 9.2 to require almost 500 cases per group, or 1000 subjects in all. The numbers of subjects required to detect even quite large differences are often a great surprise to the potential trialist. Tversky and Kahneman (1971) have conducted a study in which they found that many investigators have an exaggerated belief in the value of small amounts of data. They found that the typical believer in the value of small numbers overestimated the power of small experiments; had undue confidence in early trends as seen in the first few subjects; had unreasonably high expectations about the replicability of significant results; and rarely attributed an 'unexpected' result in an experiment to sampling variation, but tended to 'explain' causally any peculiar findings. Tversky and Kahneman conclude by this last tendency that belief in the value of small numbers can remain forever intact!

Table 9.2 Numbers of subjects per group required to detect a given treatment difference (T) expressed in numbers of standard deviations for significance level = 5 per cent and power = 95 per cent (modified from Kastenbaum et al, 1970)

| T | N per group |
|---|---|
| 0.16 | 1000 |
| 0.23 | 500 |
| 0.36 | 200 |
| 0.52 | 100 |
| 0.66 | 60 |
| 0.82 | 40 |
| 0.95 | 30 |
| 1.02 | 26 |
| 1.11 | 22 |
| 1.32 | 16 |
| 1.71 | 10 |
| 2.10 | 7 |

The foregoing discussion is concerned with trials of fixed sample size, in that the number of cases to be studied is decided before data collection begins. An alternative methodology can be used in suitable circumstances. This is a method known as SEQUENTIAL ANALYSIS. A decision is made after each paired observation either to stop further data collections because the treatment difference is statistically significant or is unlikely to be as great as the desired precision of the trial, or to continue collecting more data because it is not yet possible to reach an acceptably reliable conclusion. The use of sequential analysis in medicine is clearly described by Armitage (1975). This method is most suitable for trials in which there is one major criterion of success or failure, and in which the follow-up time necessary for patient assessment is relatively short in comparison with the recruitment rate. In suitable circumstances a sequential trial will, on average, require fewer patients than a fixed sample size trial of equal sensitivity, significance level and power.

It is most important that informal 'data snooping' is not carried out. The two statistically valid options are to use a fixed sample size determined in advance, or to perform a correct sequential analysis. Data snooping, the application of significance tests to the data whenever an 'interesting' difference is seen, is analogous to watching a horse race and stopping it whenever the horse one wishes to win is ahead.

## Conclusions

A clinical trial must be carefully designed and the data collection carried out so that the measurements on the patients are RELEVANT, free from OBSERVER BIAS, and adequately ACCURATE. The experimental design should ensure the absence of unwanted CONFOUNDING, and the size of the investigation should ensure the desired PRECISION at acceptable probabilities of Type I and Type II Errors. Any departure from a fixed sample size strategy should be on the basis of a formal SEQUENTIAL ANALYSIS, and not by performing invalid 'data snooping' when 'interesting' differences appear.

REFERENCES

Armitage, P. (1975) *Sequential Medical Trials.* 2nd ed. Oxford: Blackwell Scientific Publications.
Cochran, W.G. & Cox, G.M. (1957) *Experimental Designs.* 2nd ed. New York: Wiley.
Fisher, B. (1973) Cooperative clinical trials in primary breast cancer. *Cancer,* **31,** 1271 - 1286.
Kastenbaum, M.A., Hoel, D.G. & Bowman, K.O. (1970) Sample size requirements: one-way analysis of variance. *Biometrika,* **57,** 421 - 430.
Macrae, K.D. (1969) Serial position and sequential dependencies in repeated measures designs. *Perceptual and Motor Skills,* **29,** 736 - 738.
Tversky, A. & Kahneman, D. (1971) Belief in the law of small numbers. *Psychological Bulletin,* **76,** 105 - 110.

SUGGESTIONS FOR FURTHER READING

Armitage, P. (1971) *Statistical Methods in Medical Research.* Oxford: Blackwell Scientific Publications.
Lancaster, H.O. (1974) *An Introduction to Medical Statistics.* New York: Wiley.
Remington, R.D. & Schork, M.A. (1970) *Statistics with Applications to the Biological and Health Sciences.* Englewood Cliffs: Prentice-Hall.

# Discussion Part 2

*Dr. A. Hewett (Hoechst):* Dr. Burley, is it not inadvisable to use the terms 'crossover', 'matched pairs' and 'sequential' to describe different types of clinical trials? Any two or indeed all three of the techniques can be employed in the same trial.

*Dr. Burley:* Yes, I agree with you entirely.

*Dr. T. Pulvertaft (Zyma):* You say that when answering three nominal questions - slightly better, a lot better, very much better - there is always a tendency to pick the middle one. Nobody has ever proved that this is true.

*Dr. Burley:* Yes they have. There was an example in a paper some time ago. I can not remember the reference. Four rating scales apparently showed no difference between the drug and a comparative preparation: But when all six points on a nominal rating scale were used, there was a significant difference. I can give you the illustration even if I can not find the reference.

*Dr. R.K. Rondel (Bristol-Myers):* I was greatly moved by Pastor Burley's sermon. It should only be prefaced by the ordinary phase I trial which is given in Genesis, where it says that Moses took two tablets and went up into the mountain!

I am interested in the concept which seems to be gaining ground, that there really are such things as identically matched medications. You could add to the already formidable list of Joyce the fact that patients throw things onto the fire to see if they burn the same coloured flame, and such practices. Would you say whether you really think that double blind trials of this kind can be done any more, bearing in mind the constraints of the Health Authorities, bioavailability and bioequivalence. We seem to be in a difficult situation.

*Dr. Burley:* Dr. Cromie wrote a letter recently to the *British Medical Journal* or the *Lancet* commenting on this and pointing out that there are other ways of achieving blindness in trials than being absolutely sure that the medications are identical. We really have got a problem here. Certainly you can achieve blindness by having one doctor as observer and another doctor who monitors or changes the treatment so that the person making the observations is unaware of the medication. I do not know whether anybody has actually done any trials to see whether a trial done with bad matching tablets and good matching tablets actually gives any different results. I think this has been done and I would not be surprised if the results were much the same. I think sometimes there is a preoccupation with the matching.

*Chairman:* I notice that if the first draft of the DHSS regulations for labelling tablets were followed then a double blind trial would be impossible. Do these regulations still apply?

*Dr. Burley:* I do not know whether they still apply. Judging by the recent publications, people have spent a lot of effort in code cracking. I think it is probably very difficult to match medications adequately.

*Chairman:* Dr. Downie, have the regulations now been revised?

*Dr. C.C. Downie (I.C.I.):* The situation has been pointed out to the DHSS.

*Dr. G.M. Whitford (Warner):* When we exclude certain patients, are we going too far and ending up with selective data, from which we extrapolate to the general population?

How representative are these highly selected samples with their multiple exclusions? How relevant are they to general clinical practice?

*Dr. Burley:* This is a good question and one about which I have written and am very interested. One of the criticisms, particularly of hospital trials, is that they are conducted on a very specialised group of patients. This group is not typical of the type of patients which are going to be treated with the drug in general practice. This is a strong argument for multicentre general practice trials, providing they are conducted under suitable circumstances with the correct protocol.

*Dr. C. Kratochvil (Upjohn Europe):* Mr. Grady, I would like to ask your advice or opinion on two problems:

Firstly, have you experienced difficulty or have you solved the problem of 'lag time'? This is the delay between events occurring in the field (especially in multicentre international trials) and the receipt of these events and reorganisation at headquarters. This causes concern with potent new drugs with the possibility for therapeutic misadventure.

Secondly, we have a problem with computer programmes that are designed to digest and then regurgitate masses of data at the end of a trial. How do you permit the medical monitor to assess the current progress of significant events?

*Mr. Grady:* In answer to the second question: With regard to immediate access, we can operate the service of interrogation and presentation of results. If the question has that urgency, then one can get the answers the next day. We are putting a video display unit into our system so that we will be able to interrogate the files. There are problems with this because some of the files are tucked away as economically as possible. They are not easily interrogated. The answer for immediate access is to put in a hardware system so that people can either use it themselves or sit down with an experienced operator who understands the system and understands what is going on. We see it as either direct access by the enquirer or through a specialist user of the system.

With regard to the first question, the movement of data across international boundaries; we find that data are the easiest things to move around. If the data are acceptable, the actual movement is most easily done by either sending magnetic tapes or in the slowest form, by sending packs of cards. We try to design the sheets so that there is no alignment from the record back to any particular system. We would hope that the data which we collect are in such a form that it could be used in any system in any area. It would not matter whether they were using a desk calculator or a giant IBM facility to process the data.

*Dr. B.T. Marsh (Leo):* How much involvement does the medical adviser have in the handling of your report forms? As far as I can see, once these report forms are filled in by the clinician, the medical adviser does not see them at all. He only sees the data that have been generated by these forms and analysed by your department. One aspect of the art of a medical adviser is detecting in the returned report forms any problems that have arisen. We know of one occasion in the last year when a doctor falsified reports. This was detected by the medical adviser seeing similar writing and results on each report form.

*Mr. Grady:* We do not preclude anyone from seeing the completed reports. In some cases we put a section on the form for 'comments by Medical Department of ICI Pharmaceutical Division'. The medical adviser can look through the forms and make comments and sign them. It is not always done but there is nothing within the system to stop it being done.

*Chairman:* As a general rule, does the medical adviser see the report form when it comes back?

*Mr. Grady:* No.

*Mr. M. Ruxton (Duphar):* You mentioned that a punch card operator is like a good wife, but even good wives make a few errors. Punch card operators, no matter how good, make at least a seven per cent error. Is there any way you can reduce this?

*Mr. Grady:* I think that seven per cent is rather high. Most commercial bureaux work on a two per cent error rate. They mean, not that they will make two per cent errors, but that if you give them 100 fully punched cards, each with 96 bits of information, then there will be only two errors in 9,600 bits of information. They do operate on a claim to a much higher efficiency, but they still make mistakes. We deal with this problem whilst reading things into our computer system. We run validation programmes which will pull out the grosser types of mistake. If the recording is 83 and the girl punches 85, it will not detect that kind of error. When you set up the system you say all values between 70 and 90 are acceptable. If they make an error within the acceptable area, then there is really no way to detect it. As such the problem is insoluble.

*Dr. C.R. Lucas (Organon):* Many comments have been make about totally dissociating medical activities from marketing activities. Logistically this is impractical in most trials. Dr. Snell, you discussed clinical trials with general practitioners. When we market a new drug, we ask doctors to report side effects to the CSM. We know that they are not good at doing this. If we encourage them by any financial method, they still do not do it. If we then try to encourage them to report side effects and efficacy by calling it a clinical trial, we are accused of using this clinical trial as a marketing activity. How can we win?

*Dr. Snell:*  This is a difficult area which will always keep coming back. I can not define the difference between a commercial trial and a clinical trial; because all clinical trials or other scientific work on the drug that are favourable to it are going to have commercial implications. If it appears to be beneficial, comparative studies are set up particularly with the leading competitor. From the doctor's point of view, it is a valid comparison and therefore relevant. If drug X is widely used and you have a new drug Y, it is useful for the doctor to know how drug Y compares with drug X, apart from the commercial considerations. I think there is a clear dividing line in the organisation of clinical work depending on who does it and what their responsibilities are. If the medical department staff do it, there is a built in safeguard and a reputation for all the work. But when circulars are sent to thousands of doctors asking them to take part in a trial; when they are offered money to send back data; or when representatives call and leave cards to be filled in for a reward; then I think it is difficult to call it a scientific trial. I think the line is drawn there. The Code of Practice Committee is able to adjudicate in its particular way when required to do so on this particular question. There are a number of criteria and this is an important one. Another depends on whether the company supplies its drug free. It must do so for all proper scientific trials. If the doctor is asked to prescribe the drug on an EC10, then the 'study' is unlikely to be a clinical trial. It is much more like a marketing exercise.

*Dr. P.J. Roylance (Merck, Sharp & Dohme):*  Dr. Nicholson, there is an inflationary item whose omission may mislead some readers. If one pays for a clinical investigator in an academic unit or hospital, the appropriate salary can be determined in the back of the *British Medical Journal.* But if you work your budget on this figure you will be ten to fifteen per cent out. Certain items must be added to this salary, such as superannuation, National Health Insurance, and any number of administration charges. One therefore must not only allow for increments and inflation, but also for the sizeable trimmings.

*Dr. W.L. Burland (Smith, Kline and French):*  Dr. Nicholson, what is your opinion of those so called 'companies' not necessarily operating in general practice, who are prepared to conduct clinical studies for high costs? You did not mention these. You described the way we have been used to conducting clinical studies; but during the last year or more, there has been the appearance of what can only be called 'commercial organisations' conducting clinical trials. I am referring to a tendency for the habits of North America to spread into this country, and for certain investigators, previously rational people, appearing to think that they can charge exorbitant sums for studies.

*Dr. Nicholson:*  Yes, whether or not you use these particular organisations depends upon your needs. If I was alone in a small company with little assistance from within that company or outside, I would consider using outside help. In a large organisation such as the one in which I work, I do not think that there is generally any use for such companies. Certainly they inflate the cost of clinical trials.

*Dr. T. Pulvertaft (Zyma):*  The statistician designs a form full of little boxes with numbers on them. Take that to a clinician and he says 'Look, I asked you to make the form as simple as possible. It is going to take me all day to fill that up.' If you simplify the form by leaving off all the confusing numbers and boxes, you are left with a large white card blank except for the definition of illness. This upsets the statistician. Is there no intermediate point?

*Dr. MacRae:* I am afraid that there is not much we can do for the present generation of doctors. But we are trying to improve the standards in medical schools. We are requiring three 'A' levels, at quite a high grade now, with perhaps some quantitative ability. We hope that once these students graduate, people who find the present situation difficult can retire gracefully. Then we will have clinicians who can cope with science in its real complexity instead of artificially simplifying it!

*Chairman:* I am interested in psychiatry and believe in self examination; therefore in which of your categories do you place yourself?

*Dr. MacRae:* It depends on the phase of the moon. There is an interaction between the client and statistician. You as a psychiatrist are probably sometimes highly directive and at other times nondirective, depending on the patient. I fit my mood to the client.

*Dr. W. Bogie (Hoechst):* We unfortunately have to live in the real world. If I first take my study to a statistician, I want one who understands my problem. I am sure you are not as bullish as you appear and you probably do understand the problems: but more seriously, the problem is a very real one. Doctors think in terms of small numbers not because we are conditioned but because for practical reasons these are all the patients that are available. We have to work in small numbers and make do with small numbers. I often take my data to the statistician last because I know otherwise the sort of thing he is going to say to me, 'you can not do this, you can not do that'. But I have never yet met a statistician who can not do something with my data.

*Dr. MacRae:* Dr. Bogie, you are an excellent example of the species 'the believer in small numbers'.

# PART 3
# THE RUNNING AND EVALUATION
# OF CLINICAL TRIALS

# 10. Getting the Trial off the Ground: Logistics, Presentation of Supplies

A. W. GALBRAITH

Many of the problems concerning the evaluation of a particular therapy will always remain to be surmounted one way or another. However, advances are made in the production of medication, improvements in protocol design occur and better printing and packaging of supplies are available as a result of modern technology. These, taken with the greater experience of those responsible for the planning and execution of clinical trials, can result in better studies. It is the object of this chapter to illustrate some of the practical problems of the clinical trial and suggest ways of overcoming them.

## The protocol

This is the sheet anchor of the clinical trial and if this is not agreed amongst all the participants, the trial will founder. If the draft protocol has been accepted in principle, with dis-harmony only on minor points, there is much to be said for having a short pilot trial or dummy run. This will allow adjustment to the design and should result in the full-scale trial proceeding without difficulty.

## Lift off

For a successful launch the following should be present:

### Enthusiasm of the investigators

This is vital to the viability of the trial and it is intimately linked with the incentives of those responsible for the study. These include scientific enquiry, self advancment in a professional sense, the publication of a paper, or money. The latter may be disguised as equipment for the department or a trip to an overseas symposium but it does represent a reward for work which is time consuming, responsible and often technically difficult. In these financially stringent times, drug evaluation both at a pharmacological level and in clinical trials, can provide a realistic income for many departments, the money coming in the main from the pharmaceutical industry.

One must not forget the enthusiasm of all personnel concerned with the trial. The pharmacist, laboratory staff, radiologist, nurse, health visitor and patient, should all want the study to be a success. Check their incentives or the trial may founder.

### Good back up

In any operation, reliable, responsible advice, encouragement and resupply is necessary. Throughout the time up to and including the start of the trial, confidence in the research body, the medical adviser or the pharmaceutical company itself, will be established or lost. If the latter the trial may well be stillborn.

Although there are now ethical committees, trial certification and regulatory constraints, the competent adviser with a cooperative company should be able to produce the investigator's requirements on time.

### Stable patient situation

It is frequently noted that once a trial starts, the previously observed flow of suitable clinical material dries up. A probable explanation is that the protocol demands a strict screening of patients for inclusion which eliminates a high proportion of patients considered suitable under less critical scrutiny. It is nevertheless preferable for a trial to proceed at the planned rate to keep interest alive and to produce relevant results. This problem was illustrated during a trial of an antiepileptic drug in children having had no previous anticonvulsant treatment. The paediatric neurologist considered that at least two new cases of epilepsy were referred to him each week. This proved to be true but in most instances these were selected patients who were already resistant to conventional regimes. Another consultant, who tended to see unselected epileptics, was invited to join the trial which then went well.

### Stable staff situation

Not uncommonly a consultant will agree to carry out a trial, but as the starting date approaches, the registrar or house officer is deputed to do the work. The junior staff may be interested but if enthusiasm for the project is lacking, the trial may well not even start. It must also be remembered that if one registrar agrees to perform the study, his successor may not.

Once should also remember that there may be a delay of six months or more between the conception of a trial and the starting date. Staff whose cooperation will have already been obtained may change, so constant liaison with the different departments concerned with the study is essential. The same principles apply to trials in general practice where a change of doctor, receptionist or secretary may delay the start of the study. Sickness and leave should also be taken into account with the provision of deputies where necessary.

### Stable 'political' situation

At times of industrial tension, additional work such as a clinical trial tends to be shelved. Strikes, 'go slows' and work to rule, although uncommon in the health sector, are seen more frequently than before. Fortunately such action tends to be short lived, so any study may only be delayed briefly.

### Logistics

This is a military term meaning movement and supply which applies equally well to the civilian sector. Good planning anticipates problems, be it for a hospital or general practice, single or multicentre trial.

The closer the hospital is to the organizer's office, the cheaper and easier are planning and supply. Any problems which delay the start of a study can be handled personally rather than by letter or telephone.

Screening body fluids to assess function and drug levels becomes more commonly expected in clinical trials. The collection, storage, despatch and ultimate estimation of these fluids may pose problems. Collection may be frequent, storage may be at a specified temperature, despatch may be under special conditions and estimation may be at a centre remote from the trial centre. Personal delivery, the post, air or rail transport (each service stipulates special conditions relating to the carriage of pathological specimens) and commercial delivery services can be used. One enterprising family doctor arranged with the local bus company that a vacuum flask containing swabs which he left at a certain bus stop was to be picked up by the conductor and deposited at the ambulance station en route. The next ambulance travelling to the hospital delivered the flask to the laboratory, fifteen miles from the doctor's surgery.

For the smooth progress of any trial, it helps if the organizer is kept informed right from the start how it is going. In the large multicentre study this is particularly important. One method is to code number each patient entering the trial, post a card to the organizer informing him that this number has been taken up and report when this individual drops out or completes the study. Stocks of record forms, medication, test equipment or other necessary items can thus be maintained.

Careful planning, attention to detail and, if necessary, a dummy run should ensure a prompt start and a smoothly progressive investigation.

## Presentation of supplies

Although many excellent trials are performed using simple duplicated record sheets and tablets counted from bulk in outpatients, mistakes can occur more easily under such circumstances. Clearly printed, colour coded record forms and prepacked code labelled containers holding the correct quantity of medication, will do much to eliminate inaccuracy and promote efficiency in a study.

Attractively presented material can be reassuring both to the clinician and the patient. An illustration of the improvement in a kit which was supplied to general practitioners for a trial of an antiviral agent is shown in Figures 10.1 and 10.2. The first was used in 1970 and required boxes made specially to contain the large record forms. The second used attractively constructed boxes originally produced in bulk to hold cosmetic samples. The record forms were scaled to fit these cheaper but superior containers.

The mode of presentation of medication, be it in capsules, tablets, syrup, cream, suppositories or ampoules for injection, requires careful thought. A placebo controlled single drug trial in hospital, for example, is probably best done through the pharmacy using the standard containers.

### Strip or blister packing

If strip or blister packing is indicated, the medication is most conveniently prepared by the pharmaceutical company. One of the advantages of strip packing over individual containers lies in the ability to pack tablets of one composition along one

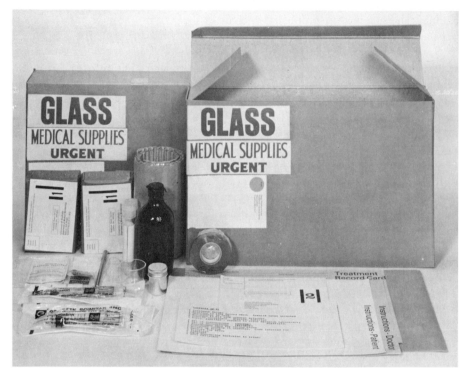

Fig. 10.1  Trial Kit, Mark I, 1970

side and tablets of an identical looking placebo along the other. Stapling or glueing the strip in printed catch covers enables a double-dummy design to be employed without having to dispense the tablets in the much less elegant twin containers.

A variable dosage scheme may be employed with strip packing using identical looking tablets containing different amounts of drug. The catch covers in this trial design must be accurately identified by the pharmacist and the dosage regime be absolutely clear to the patient. The blister pack has been successfully used by the manufacturers of the sequential contraceptive pill. If trial medication is to be taken in a particular order, this is an ideal method of presentation.

### Placebo

The composition of the placebo may give rise to concern. It is usually considered necessary to present this as an item indistinguishable from the active preparation (Anderson, Ashley and Clarke, 1976) but this need not be the case (Cromie, 1976). It would seem sensible that in double blind or single blind trials the test substances should be in as near identical form as possible. Doctor and patient will hazard a guess on the composition. If the medication is correctly identified, the differences between active and placebo tend to be increased while if incorrectly identified, the differences tend to be reduced.

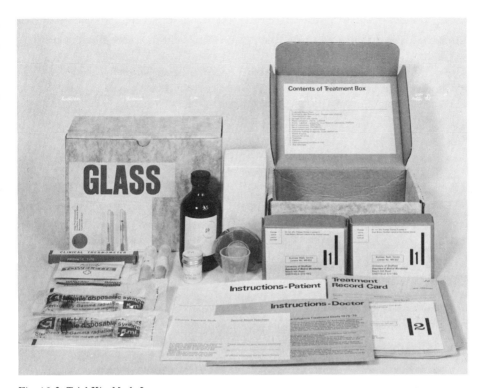

Fig. 10.2  Trial Kit, Mark 2.

*Detail*

Every step in a trial should be considered in detail. A multicentre general practitioner study of shingles based on the design for the influenza investigation, in spite of initial misgivings, worked well (Galbraith, 1973). All the equipment necessary was provided, even a small roll of sticky tape was included to seal the serum specimen box prior to postage. Time is a precious commodity and anything which can save even minutes during a trial is to be recommended.

## Conclusion

A practical protocol, an enthusiastic and settled staff, sufficient suitable patients, carefully considered logistics and a competent coordinator should result in a satisfactory start to the study.

REFERENCES

Anderson, T.W., Ashley, M.J. & Clarke, E.A. (1976) Not so double blind? *British Medical Journal,* **1**, 457 - 458.

Cromie, B.W. (1976) Not so double blind? *British Medical Journal,* **1**, 710.

Galbraith, A.W. (1973) Treatment of acute Herpes zoster with amantadine hydrochloride (Symmetrel). *British Medical Journal,* **4**, 693 - 695.

# 11. Keeping the Trial Going: Medical Advisers or Coordinators; Prescription Costs

B. T. MARSH

There are really three sections to this chapter, namely:
1. What are medical advisers?
2. What should they do when the trial is running?
3. Who pays for the drugs?

Clearly, as a medical adviser in the pharmaceutical industry, I will try to answer these questions from the industry point of view. However, many of the principles defined in the second section on 'Keeping the Trial Going' are equally applicable to any physician brave enough, or mad enough, to agree to set up and coordinate a clinical trial. There should be no basic differences between a study set up by a physician working in the pharmaceutical industry and one set up by a physician in hospital or general practice. The reasons for the studies and their organisation and running should be equally ethical and efficient. If they are not, then the organiser is performing a disservice both to his profession and to himself.

## Role of medical adviser

Let us look first at the role of the medical adviser in the various aspects of keeping a trial going. A perusal of the literature reveals varying definitions of his function such as:

Adviser
Coordinator
Trouble shooter
Interpreter
Link man
Monitor
Supervisor
Efficient clerk
'Dogsbody'

There is no one word that truly describes the role of the medical adviser. This list illustrates that he is all things to all men, which is probably as it should be. In the last symposium on the Principles and Practice of Clinical Trials, Galbraith (1970) put it rather more succinctly. He said that the medical adviser could be a useful link man:

Chivvying the consultant
Fortifying the family physician
Pacifying the pharmacist

Liaising with the laboratory

Solacing the secretary

The difficulties in clearly defining the medical adviser's role can now be seen: He is the proverbial 'Jack of all trades'. Despite extensive planning and preparation, unforeseen problems will always arise in trials. The medical adviser must be able to modify, relabel, repack, reprint or do whatever is appropriate to overcome the snags and get the trial going again. He may need to provide some stimulant or motivation to restart a trial that has drifted into the doldrums due to waning interest, change of staff or other reasons (Cromie, 1973). Finally, he may need to drastically modify or even stop the study if unacceptable side effects or adverse reactions appear during the course of the investigation. At the same time he must ensure that all personnel involved are informed of any changes and steps taken to ensure adequate follow up of patients. All these problems must be overcome at the same time as retaining the confidence and respect of the investigator.

Can we define his role any further? The only word that comes anywhere near the true function is 'governor'; not in its governmental connotation or Cockney usage, but in its mechanical meaning. This is 'automatic regulator of supply of gas, steam, water, etc. to machine, ensuring even motion.' Substitute motivation, materials and aid for gas, steam and water, and trial for machine, and you have something near the ideal definition.

**Keeping the trial going**

It is impossible to discuss the ways and means of keeping a trial going without emphasising the need for careful and meticulous planning before it even starts. Over 90 per cent of the potential causes of trial failure can and should be anticipated in this stage, and appropriate steps taken to avoid them.

Harris (1966) defined nine phases of a clinical trial:

Interest

Reading

Preliminary design

Decision

Trial design

Execution

Analysis

Assessment

Report writing

We are concerned with the 'execution', a singularly appropriate word since, if the trial does collapse, the medical adviser in charge may well end up as the sacrificial offering. Therefore, before the trial starts, the medical adviser must ensure to his full satisfaction that all of the preliminary work and planning is adequate. The protocol and instructions for the investigators and ancillary staff must be read carefully and with the eye of a doubter. That is, try and find any statement or instruction that can be misread or is equivocal. If any instruction can be misunderstood, it will be sooner or later. Run through the arrangements for supplying the clinical trial materials, the reporting system, and delivery of samples. Is there a weak link? If there is one, be sure it will be discovered. An excellent way to discover potential problem areas is to have a pilot trial before the main study begins. This is particularly important in the large scale multicentre studies, or in the long term studies, but is equally useful in other trials until your technique has been validated in active service.

It is essential to have a firm understanding of the basic principles and not clutter up one's thoughts with sophisticated techniques and ploys. These can come later as you gain experience in clinical trial methodology and become aware of the areas in which trouble most often occurs. In the meantime, someone else will have used the latest new technique, if you are lucky, and reported on its shortcomings. You can then decide at leisure on whether it is a worthwhile advance.

There are six  basic principles to follow when running a trial, namely:
Preparation
Cooperation
Attestation
Administration
Dissemination
Anticipation

## Preparation

This area has been covered more than adequately in previous chapters. However, it must be emphasised once again that the most important part of any study is the preparation. Once a study is in progress, any fault that occurs will be magnified out of all proportion to its size and take a disproportionate amount of time and effort to correct.

## Cooperation

Cooperation with, and cultivation of, the people involved in a study is time-consuming, sometimes frustrating and occasionally troublesome on the digestion. What it is not, is a waste of time. The main investigator will need a full briefing on the study, together with his colleagues to whom the work may be delegated. But how often are the ward sisters or the nurses in the unit given a briefing on the aims and objects of the study? When was the last time you actually met any of the nurses who had to collect and forward to the laboratory the 24 hour urine samples that were an essential element of your study?

If you are investigating an antibiotic, the consultant microbiologist and physician will be briefed on the various assay techniques to be used. Have you thought of the technician who will be plating out the organism and taking the readings? Does he know the object of the study and how important it is to perform the assays as soon as he receives the specimens and not to freeze them to perform at leisure later? Who says 'well done' when he gets the specimens at 4.30 p.m. and stays on until the work is completed?

Time spent in finding out their names and meeting these important cogs in the trial programme is well worthwhile, and often a lesson only learnt by bitter experience. This does not only apply to those at the trial centre. Many departments in the pharmaceutical company may be involved, not all of them medical. When you sign an order for a rush despatch of clinical trial materials, do you know how that order will be processed and how long it will take for the parcels to get to the railway station or post office? Do you know the name of the person who will have to slog up to the railway station at 5.30 p.m. to ensure that it gets on the next train to Newcastle or wherever it may be? All this may seem extremely tedious and unnecessary. But do not forget there may be several rush orders or late arrivals of samples requiring immediate analysis. The best way to ensure continuation of the study is to get to know these people and to ensure that their efforts are appreciated.

### Attestation

Not a beautiful word, but one that defines this principle. Much of the testing of procedures will have been performed during the planning stages or in the pilot study. A continual watch during the course of the study is still required if you are to avoid a deterioration in the quality of work or provision of information. The staff at the trial centre may become ill, go on holiday or be transferred. Locums are often dropped into a trial situation without any information on the aims, objects and procedures. Frequent checks on these points will allow you to monitor any changes and provide advice or help before it is too late.

The nursing procedures and laboratory investigations also need regular attestation. It is surprising how often changes in ward routine occur in the middle of your trial. Similarly, why is it that the autoanalyser always breaks down in your study or the microbiological laboratory discovers a contaminant organism in your plates? These things do occur, and if you can recount such instances, it does show you were aware that they had happened. What is inexcusable is a change in ward routine or laboratory techniques of which the medical adviser is unaware, with the resulting change in baseline parameters.

In a multicentre study, frequent visits to all the centres will check that the interviewing, assessment and recording of data is consistent. This is a more difficult problem than it would first appear. Similarly, try and ensure that there are enough checks on patient compliance and acceptance of medication. We make the presumption that provided we design our study correctly and the appropriate treatment is offered to the correct patient under the proper conditions, all will be well. Very often it is not. Many studies have shown that between 15 and 52 per cent of patients are not taking their treatment. You would not know this unless you took steps to find out (Maxwell, 1973). There is no absolutely reliable method for checking that patients have taken their medication. However, if the early results of the study are anomalous, or the investigator suddenly loses enthusiasm, a check on patient acceptance of medication is always worthwhile. There is an indirect way that you can check on patient compliance. You may know from past experience the type of side effect or adverse reaction to expect from the drug in question. A quick glance at the section recording side effects will show whether the expected numbers are appearing.

Regular examination of the clinical trial material and analysis of drug samples is a wise precaution. Pilot production batches of material may show unequal colour or consistency changes after a variable period of time (Galbraith, 1970). Active intervention may not be necessary, although any gross changes, despite normal potency, may introduce unacceptable bias. Remember also that placebos can also change in colour or consistency. In a double blind study, keep a constant watch on 'the guessing game' of deciding which is the active or standard drug since even a wrong guess can bias the clinical evaluation. These are a few of the areas needing constant supervision. The occasional surprise visits ensure that you know what is happening or where problems might arise.

## Administration

There can be few excuses on the part of a medical adviser if the administration of a study breaks down. It is his job to see that there is sufficient expertise at both his end and that of the trial centre. This is where cultivation and a few kind words and smiles can bring their rewards.

Is there someone with sufficient knowledge of the study to stand in for you when you are away or ill? Are the case records being duplicated as they arrive or is there a copy at the trial centre? Sooner or later a keen secretary or office cleaner is going to shred or throw away that pile of paper gathering dust on the table or bookcase. With the postal service as it is, duplication of records at source is a wise precaution if possible.

Other aspects of administration include the mastering of the paperwork involved in ordering supplies, instruments, equipment and their despatch to the people needing them. Payments for various parts of the study may be necessary at regular intervals. Accountants have an annoying habit of trying to save the company money. They do this by collecting all your memos requesting payment over the past three months and providing you with the appropriate cheques in one go. This way they gain interest on the cash involved. Praiseworthy though this may be, it is not the excuse you should give to your trialist when he asks why his grant is ten weeks overdue. Make sure you know where the company accountant works; ask about his family and give the occasional advice on minor medical matters. This usually works wonders when you ask him not to delay payment to any of your trialists!

Basically, administration comes down to the simple principle of keeping people informed and making provision for the times when you are not available.

## Dissemination

To continue with the horticultural analogy, dissemination is part of cultivation. Just as there is a need to visit the trial centre and meet the investigators, there is also the need to keep all the personnel involved up to date with any information relevant to the study. Again, do not forget the paramedical staff and your colleagues in your company. Let them know that the study is progressing satisfactorily and that their efforts are appreciated and worthwhile.

In a long term study or in a multicentre trial, information sheets sent round at regular intervals are a useful means of disseminating information and keeping everyone in the picture. Periodical meetings may be useful, although there is always the problem of getting all the interested parties together in the right place at the right time.

## Anticipation

The last principle is the art of anticipation. Many problems or potential problems can be anticipated in the planning stages and contingency plans worked out, but it is the unexpected problem arising in the middle of a study that causes the greatest upset and danger of failure. An inbuilt sixth sense is invaluable in this situation, but unfortunately it is usually only by bitter experience that this sixth sense can be developed and reinforced.

Look for the incompletely or sloppily filled in report forms. Look for the tables of laboratory results that are either too perfect or grossly incomplete. Take heed when you start having difficulties in contacting the investigator on the phone or your letters are unanswered. If you do start having doubts, the previous groundwork in visiting the trial centre and contacting the staff involved should now pay off. You will at least have some background knowledge against which to evaluate your doubts and the number of possible courses of action will be greater.

There is little more one can say about anticipation; you either develop this art or you do not. In case you are feeling complacent and recalling to yourself those occasions on which you successfully anticipated a problem, let me give a word of warning. There may be times when you feel you are more of a detective than a medical adviser, and the continual checking and cross checking may seem both useless and obnoxious. Do not forget that every trial organiser has a duty to the patient, the investigators, himself and to the company. He must try to ensure that the study is performed in an ethical and safe manner and successfully concluded if possible, no matter what the final result may be. You may feel that I am labouring this point, but let me quote from a report by the F.D.A., who investigated American physicians undertaking new drug trials. Over a three month period, 20 per cent of these physicians were guilty of a range of unethical practices, such as:

Overdosing

Underdosing

Falsifying records and consent forms

Dumping drugs in dustbins

Supposedly treating patients although the physician was on an extended vacation in Europe

Unsubstantiated laboratory reports

Concurrent administration of drugs invalidating the study

Failing to record concurrent illnesses and diseases having a bearing on the study

I cannot confirm the authenticity of this report, but I do know that such things can also happen in this country. It is part of the role of the medical adviser to be aware of these possibilities. If he does not pick them up, then the fault lies almost as much with him as with the investigator.

### Prescription costs

I should like to say a few words about prescription costs or, to put it more bluntly, who pays for what. This problem may arise at any time, but particularly when comparing a new drug against a standard drug in the premarketing phase, or comparing marketed drugs, the so called phase IV study. I am afraid that there is no simple answer since every situation is different and the costs of materials can vary widely. We are all aware of the financial pressures in regard to prescription costs, both in hospital and in general practice, As a general rule, if a company sets up a study, then it should supply its own product free of charge. I say 'as a general rule', because it is possible that a company may be unwilling to proceed with a highly expensive treatment for a rare condition, unless it could at least recover the cost of the materials used. Any decision on such charges would have to be discussed with the investigators and the reasons fully explained.

Greater difficulties arise when you wish to compare with or add to a standard drug regime which would be administered whether or not there was a clinical trial. Should you pay for the standard material or not? It depends upon the study. If repackaging and relabelling are required, or the study is double blind, then all costs should be borne by the company. If the standard regime is being given on an open basis, the payment for this material must depend upon discussions with the investigators and any others involved, such as the hospital pharmacist. If a study is really necessary and will provide useful information, you should be prepared to cover the costs of all the drugs used if they are directly involved in that study.

This chapter may appear to be too basic and to merely list some of the obvious factors involved in monitoring clinical trials. In my experience, it is a lack of appreciation of these basic principles that makes many clinical trials so difficult to manage and successfully conclude. It is only rarely that a problem arises which, in retrospect, could not have been anticipated or the study so arranged that it coped with these hiccups in its stride.

However, at some time or other we all reach the stage at which a study looks like folding up, despite all our efforts. What can be done? Probably very little, but sometimes it helps to express one's disappointment in a cogent manner. Whilst preparing this chapter, I happened to glance at an AMAPI booklet. I noticed that there was a coat of arms or insignia on the cover, no larger than a postage stamp. I am assured that the central object is a test tube, although for one moment I thought that it was a finger covered by a finger stall. With a flash of inspiration, I jotted down a motto for all medical advisers and clinical trial organisers that perhaps can be used as a last effort to get the study moving again:

'PRO DEO GRATIAS, EXTRACTUM FLAMMUM DIGITUM'

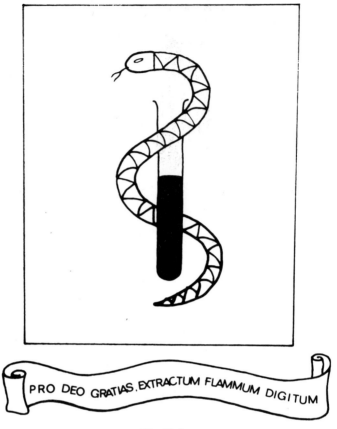

Fig 11.1

## REFERENCES

Cromie, B.W. (1973) In *International Aspects of Drug Evaluation and Usage.* ed.
  Jouhar, A.J. & Grayson, M.F. Chapter 16 pp. 171 - 176, Edinburgh & London:
  Churchill Livingstone.
Galbraith, A.W. (1970) In *The Principles and Practice of Clinical Trials.* ed. Harris,
  E.L. & Fitzgerald, J.D. Part I, pp. 106 - 111, Edinburgh & London: Churchill
  Livingstone.
Harris, E.L. (1966) The clinical trial in general practice. *Journal of College of General
  Practitioners,* **12,** 43 - 53.
Maxwell, C. (1973) *Clinical Research for All.* Cambridge Medical Publications Ltd.,
  Northampton.

# 12. Adverse Reaction Monitoring

A. W. HARCUS

An adverse drug reaction has been described as any event that follows the administration of a drug given in the recommended dose, is atrributable to the administration of that drug and is harmful to the recipient, the foetus she carries or, by an effect on the gonads, to the recipient's descendants (Doll, 1972).

This definition differentiates adverse reactions which are harmful and occur at the recommended dose from toxic effects which are harmful and result from doses in excess of the therapeutic range and also from side effects which need not necessarily be harmful.

Detection and assessment of undesirable effects is just as important in the development of a new compound as the objective evaluation of beneficial effects. It is estimated that between five and ten per cent of admissions to hospital medical wards are a result of adverse reactions to drugs administered outside hospital. A complete profile of the drug must be built up, for it is only when the risk to benefit ratio has been determined that the physician can compare the advantages and disadvantages before prescribing appropriate therapy for his patient. Moderately severe adverse reactions, for example, may be quite acceptable in life threatening situations whereas they would be totally unacceptable in the treatment of minor ailments.

Some adverse reactions can be confidently predicted from knowledge of the chemical, pharmacological or metabolic properties of the compound. Many are totally unexpected and may be quite rare which makes detection by conventional clinical trial methods extremely unlikely.

Techniques for detecting adverse reactions differ, therefore, from those used for the evaluation of beneficial effects. The W.H.O. has defined adverse reactions monitoring as any procedure that aims at providing systematic inferences on likely chains of causation linking drugs and adverse reactions within a population (W.H.O., 1972).

Information about undesirable effects can be collected by intensive surveillance of a defined population, from spontaneous reports or by means of record linkage and it may be prospective or retrospective. Each of the types of information and methods of collection has advantages and disadvantages. In each, careful evaluation and interpretation of the data are necessary in order to establish a true relationship between an adverse reaction and the drug.

## Record linkage

A comprehensive medical history of individual patients and the therapy they receive can be collated from a number of sources such as general practitioners, clinics, hospital out-patient departments and wards; and eventually the Registrar General who will provide details of the cause of death. Record linkage of this type is really only possible in areas with an integrated health service and adequate computer facilities. A few pilot schemes have been started both in this country and in Scandinavia. Their progress will be watched with interest because the method affords an excellent opportunity for monitoring delayed and long term reactions to drugs. This may be the only way, for instance, by which it is possible to determine the relationship between drugs and cancers developing later in life.

### Intensive surveillance

Information can be obtained about the nature and incidence of adverse reactions to drugs and the extent to which they are prescribed by intensive surveillance of a discrete population. Surveys of this type are usually restricted to patients in hospital but have occasionally been conducted on a regional basis.

The drawbacks of hospital monitoring are that the pattern of prescribing may differ considerably from that encountered in general practice, the patients are generally more severely ill and are probably exposed to a greater number and variety of drugs. The total population available for study is limited and the cost of recording, extracting and processing information is likely to be high in comparison with some other methods of monitoring.

Reliable and detailed information can be collected about the patients, the drugs they are taking and the undesirable effects they experience. With this knowledge, specific groups of patients at risk such as those with a history of allergy, or the elderly, can be identified and retrospective data from the programme can be easily examined in order to follow up and investigate spontaneous reports of adverse reactions. If necessary prospective studies can then be undertaken to clarify the situation and to confirm or refute the association between the reaction and the drug.

The better known intensive surveillance programmes are those in Boston, USA and Aberdeen. The Boston Collaborative Drug Surveillance Programme was established in 1966 to measure the efficacy and toxicity of drugs used in hospital, to detect unsuspected drug effects, to investigate interactions and to evaluate genetic and acquired patient characteristics which influence drug effects. Data from medical, paediatric and psychiatric wards of eleven hospitals are monitored. The connection between a drug and an adverse reaction is expressed on a four point scale as definite, probable, doubtful or don't know. Jick (1972) has reported that in 4.8 per cent of all drug exposures, there was an adverse reaction which was possibly or probably drug induced.

The Medicines Evaluation and Monitoring Group has been collecting information about drugs used in Aberdeen hospitals for eight years. It has a record of about one million prescriptions for some 250,000 patients, indexed by age, sex, diagnosis and drug. Recent studies have included investigations into the possible association of rauwolfia derivatives with breast cancer and that between beta blockers and the oculocutaneous syndrome. Comprehensive analysis on prescribing practices are undertaken and various aspects of drug epidemiology are currently being studied (Moir, 1976

### Spontaneous reporting

Spontaneous reporting is extremely useful as an early warning system for potential adverse reactions. It has the great advantage that rare events can be detected because vast numbers of patients from all sectors of the community are available for screening.

Reports of suspected reactions appear from time to time in the columns of the medical journals but isolated events may be misleading. Reference to a central agency is preferable if suspicions about a drug are to be confirmed or refuted. There are national and international registers for this purpose and pharmaceutical companies maintain comprehensive files on their own products.

The significance of a reaction is not necessarily reflected in the number of reports received. The reported incidence of reactions may vary widely from one drug to another depending on factors such as general awareness of potential untoward effects or publicity. It is often possible, nevertheless, to establish a profile for a drug or group of drugs from which valid conclusions can be drawn. This is clearly demonstrated by the profiles of four anti-inflammatory agents, phenylbutazone, oxyphenbutazone, indomethacin and ibufenac (Fig. 12.1). Although the patterns of reactions are quite

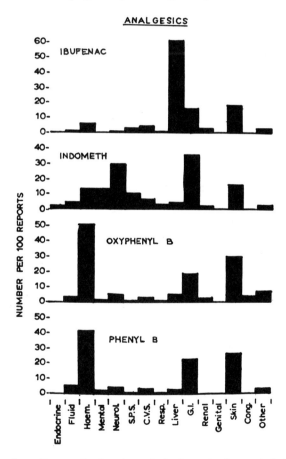

Fig. 12.1 Profiles of reactions: analgesics. An analysis of reports of suspected adverse reactions to drugs received by the Committee of Safety of Drugs between 1964 and 1969.

different the incidence of hepatic effects is considerably higher with ibufenac than with the other three products. So many reports of jaundice, hepatic necrosis and impairment of hepatic function were received by the Committee on Safety of Drugs, that it was withdrawn from the market after only three months.

The major disadvantage of spontaneous monitoring is that notification of a suspected reaction depends upon the motivation of individual clinicians; under reporting is inevitable.

Inman (1972) has estimated for instance that less than 10 per cent of the reactions in this country are actually reported to the Register of Adverse Reactions which was set up in 1964 by the Committee on Safety of Drugs. Even at this very low level of reporting it has proven impossible for the Committee to follow up every case and they have given some guidance as to the types of reactions which should be notified (C.S.M, 1972). They wish to be informed about all reactions to a new drug, however trivial, but only unusual or serious reactions to well established drugs should be reported. Included in the latter are anaphylaxis, blood dyscrasias, congenital abnormalities, electrolyte disturbances, severe CNS effects, haemorrhage, jaundice, ophthalmic signs and symptoms and severe skin reactions.

## World Health Organisation

The Register of Adverse Reactions in the UK is one of many national registries. In 1962 the Director General of the WHO was requested to initiate a programme for the promotion of the safety and efficacy of drugs. In 1968 a Research Centre for International Drug Monitoring was established to collaborate with National Centres. The WHO centre has developed systems for recording, storing, linking and retrieving reports. It has prepared a standardised terminology of adverse reactions and regularly distributes details of adverse reactions to National Centres. The value of spontaneous reporting as an early warning system has been recognised and special signals have been built into the programme to alert the monitors automatically to new reactions or increases in the reporting rate. Should these appear to be relevent, retrospective or prospective studies can be undertaken to investigate and prove or disprove a causal relationship between the drug and suspected adverse effect (Royall and Venulet, 1972).

## Pharmaceutical industry

It is also by means of spontaneous reports that those of us in the pharmaceutical industry generally learn about the unwanted effects of our drugs. The holder of a product licence has a statutory obligation 'to maintain a record of reports, of which he is aware, of adverse effects in one or more human beings or animals associated in those reports with the use of any medicinal product to which the licence relates', and to produce the records for inspection if requested (Medicines Regulations, 1971). The industry has a distinct advantage over the other agencies in the field of adverse reaction monitoring. The resources of each company are concentrated on relatively few products and the expertise of a multi-disciplinary team of scientists closely associated with the product and its development can be called upon for detailed, in-depth examination of any problems that may arise.

The importance of meticulous monitoring of both untoward and desirable effects has already been stressed. There is no better opportunity for this than in the early phases of clinical development when all supplies of the drug are completely controlled by the medical adviser and each patient can be thoroughly supervised. Care must be taken to record all effects during clinical trials and not to discard, as fortuitous, those which are unexpected or trivial. It is essential to recognise adverse reactions for what they are because subsequent interpretation will depend upon the quantity and quality of information available for assessment.

The nature and frequency of reporting is influenced by the method of approach and the kind of question asked. The response to direct questions is usually greater than to indirect questions, sometimes resulting in over reporting and the erroneous association of chance effects with a drug under investigation. No matter how carefully we monitor during clinical trials, the number and duration of exposures to the drug are limited until it becomes generally available. It is only in widespread use that the rarer reactions will occur and can be detected. There is a place for continued surveillance after launch for the first two or three years to establish a more accurate profile.

Pharmaceutical companies are ultimately responsible for the safety of their products and cannot afford merely to await events. Every effort should be made to discover the nature, cause and incidence of adverse reactions. A much more aggressive attitude to these problems should be adopted. Many larger organisations which have already set up sections within the medical departments for this purpose find they have a sounder knowledge of their products as a result.

Compilation of a clinical data base should begin the day a new compound is first given to man. An efficient retrieval system, either manual or electronic, should be designed and the world literature should be scrutinised regularly for reports about the product or closely related compounds. Reports of side effects should be followed up by correspondence or in serious cases by a visit from one of the company's physicians. In the majority of cases the findings will be inconclusive. In some cases a rechallenge may be ethically acceptable while in others additional controlled studies may be required to explore the situation fully.

### Prospective and retrospective information

The information collected by the various types of monitoring that have been described may be retrospective or prospective.

Retrospective information is subject to uncontrolled confounding factors and may be biased by patient selections. If these limitations are taken into account it can be of great value. Evaluation of data does not depend upon future events, details of rare occurrence can be sought and detected at relatively small cost and long term effects can be observed. The association between steroid contraceptives and thromboembolism and that between aerosol inhalers and the epidemic of deaths from asthma in the sixties are good examples.

Although prospective studies are often expensive and difficult to set up they can at least be properly controlled with stratification to avoid bias. Patients can be allocated at random into groups for comparative purposes. The information gained is more likely to be reliable but may take considerably longer to collect. Attention has been drawn to the dearth of such studies in a recent review of adverse reactions by Karch and Lasagna (1975).

## Conclusion

In the last decade, awareness of the need for a better comprehension of the effects of therapeutic substances has grown. As a consequence greater efforts have been made to determine both the desirable and undesirable effects of drugs. Different methods have been devised for monitoring adverse reactions. Whatever the approach, careful observation and record keeping are essential to establish a causal relationship between drug and effect, if such a relationship exists. Constant vigilance is required to ensure the detection of unwanted effects.

Our Association devoted an entire symposium in 1971 to Adverse Reactions, Their Prediction, Detection and Assessment. Those who wish to learn more about the subject will find the published proceedings an excellent starting point for further study.

REFERENCES

C.S.M. (1972) Importance of reporting adverse drug reactions. *Adverse Drug Reaction Bulletin,* **33,** 103.

Doll, W.R.S. (1972) *Adverse Drug Reactions.* Ed. Richards, D.J. & Rondel, R.K. London: Churchill Livingstone.

Inman, W.H.W. (1972) *ibid.* ch. 11 pp 86 - 101.

Jick H. (1972) *ibid.* ch. 8. pp 61 - 66.

Karch, F.E. & Lasagna, L. (1975) Adverse Drug Reactions. *J. Amer. med. Ass.,* **234,** 1236 - 1241.

Medicines (Standard Provisions for Medicines and Certificates) Regulations (1971) *S.I. No. 972.* Schedule 1, Part 1, 4. London: H.M.S.O.

Moir, D.C. (1976) *Personal Communication.*

Royall, B.W. & Venulet, J. (1972) Methodology for International Drug Monitoring. *Methods of Information of Medicine,* **11,** 2, 75 - 86.

W.H.O. (1972) International drug monitoring: the role of national centres. *W.H.O. Technical Report Series.* No. 498.

FURTHER READING

C.S.M. (1976) *Committee on Safety of Medicines: Register of Adverse Reactions.* London: D.H.S.S.

Martin, E.W. (1971) *Hazards of Medication.* Philadelphia: Lippincott.

Medicine in the Public Interest (1974) Adverse drug reactions in the United States: an analysis of the scope of the problems and recommendations for future approaches. *Medicine in the Public Interest.*

Meyler, L. (1973) *Side Effects of Drugs.* Amsterdam: Elsevier, 8.

Richards, D.S. & Rondel, R.K. (1972) *Adverse Drug Reactions.* London: Churchill Livingstone.

Stockley, I. (1974) *Drug. Interactions and their Mechanisms.* London: Pharmaceutical Press.

# 13.  Handling Data of Trial Results

F. GRADY

All the data created by clinical and field trials at ICI Pharmaceuticals Division are handled by packages. Although this statement includes the more complex technical statistics, statistical evaluation is outside the scope of data handling in this context. By data handling we mean data input, validation, edit and amendment as the initial steps in clinical trial data base compilation. The major aspects of data record handling are record manipulation, multifacet correlations, data interrelationships, data base interrogation and retrieval, and result tabulation and presentation.

All this work is done using the two ICL (International Computers Limited) software packages, SURVEY ANALYSIS and FIND-2. Our investigations since 1962 have demonstrated to us that the best approach to clinical trials is via software packages rather than specific suites of programmes.

We commenced our activities in the clinical trial information area in 1962 after long experience in chemical and biological information work. One thing quickly became apparent. In the chemical and biological areas no one knew the answers. In clinical trials no one even knew the questions. The first trial in which my group became involved was a multicentre cholesterol level lowering trial. What we did not know was how quickly this drug would lower cholesterol levels, in whom, and at what dose level. In the event cholesterol levels fell sharply at commencement of therapy in both the drug and placebo groups, although somewhat more in the drug group. Levels in both groups then rose slowly, with that of the drug patients levelling off at a reduced cholesterol level, whilst that of the placebo patients continued to rise back to pretreatment levels. We found 'seasonal variation' with patients having an upsurge of cholesterol levels twice a year. We found a group of hard core non responders. We were given to believe that the 'normal' cholesterol level was 220 mgs. We designed an elaborate cholesterol reduction index, compared the recorded levels with the 'norm' of 220 and presented the data back as a percentage improvement table. We found patients with positive percentage changes of many thousands and others with similar negative percentage changes. Investigation revealed that some patients were below the 220 level at onset and of these some went higher and some went lower. This trial did demonstrate that our drug reduced cholesterol levels. It also demonstrated that we had not answered the basic question of whether in reducing cholesterol levels we were also keeping people alive longer. It was two trials and several years later that the answers to that question emerged (Trial of Clofibrate, 1971; Ischaemic heart disease, 1971).

In a trial with a B-blocker in intensive care, the problem was that we did not know how any improvement would become apparent between the drug and placebo groups. Would more die in intensive care, would some patients require less time in intensive care would fewer need to return to intensive care, would less nursing care be required, less therapy, would some return home earlier than others, would some return to work before others, would some re-enter hospital, would some die earlier after discharge than others? And if these differences were present, who would follow which path?

In the current trial in intermittent claudication to which I referred in chapter 6, the same problems remain. We are convinced that the patients taking the drug have lowered levels of fibrinogen and viscosity, but these are laboratory measurements. It is of little relevance to the patient that the sheer rate at $0.77^{-1}$ has gone down from 37.3 to 28.5. The crux of the matter is much more mundane. If the drug is going to be beneficial to the patient, how will this benefit be demonstrated?

The possibilities which form the answer to this question are infinite, a few examples are: Will the distance a person can walk after six months on therapy compared with the distance a person can walk at entry improve? This seemingly direct yardstick is notoriously fallible with differences being due to factors such as mood, weather and temperament. Are the number of amputations in the drug group opposed to the placebo group meaningful? Is the presence or absence of gangrene in either the drug or placebo group attributable to the therapy? Does the drug act differently in people with previous reconstructive arterial surgery compared to those people without? What is the significance of concurrent drug therapy? How much easier is it to live with the condition after therapy, is the pain less severe, is the onset meaningfully later, is the patient still housebound, can he or she now walk to the local shops or the pubs? Do patients in the early stages of the disease respond differently to the more chronic cases?

Questions like these usually evolve only during the conduct of the trial. The clinician is not able to specify a full list of questions or specify the full likelihood of data interrelationship prior to the trial. This means that he is unable to specify his requirements in the usual computer programme specification context. Accordingly, the system available to him must provide post-coordination as opposed to pre-coordination facilities. Questions evolve during the conduct of the trial and the evaluation of the data. It is neither practicable to have programmers allocated to the project to reprogram as the questions emerge, nor is the length of time required to write a program acceptable to the clinician as he waits for the answers.

We found the solution to these problems in the joint development with ICL of a sophisticated punched card machine, the ICL 335 Census Statistical Sorter. This machine has facilities for sorting, counting, classification and data presentation. Latterly we have used the SURVEY ANALYSIS and FIND-2 software packages. Basically these packages are pigeonhole frameworks with flexible sides, shapes and sizes to each hole. The packages supply almost unlimited facilities to manipulate the pigeonholes. The user specifies what data he wants to go into each pigeonhole and also the size and shape of the data. For example, data could be specified as a six field entry with the first two fields for the day, related and ranging from 01 to 31, the next two for the month, related and ranging from 01 to 12, and the last two for the year, relating and ranging from 00 - 99. Where ambiguity could arise over the year of birth the field would be extended to four and cover, perhaps, 1870 to 1976.

## Survey analysis

This is a general package suitable for any application with the necessity to collect and analyse considerable quantities of accurate and relevant data about the members of any group. We have successfully adopted it in the clinical trials information sector. The overall technique of survey analysis falls naturally into three parts:

The collection of the data via well designed forms aimed at eliciting clear and unambiguous answers;

The computer analysis of this data which may occur in such large quantities as to make any other method of data handling impracticable, or of such complexity that predetermined criteria must be rigorously applied in order to obtain correct evaluations;

The interpretation of the machine coordinated data which must remain the responsibility of the clinician. Methods of analysis and presentation of data must be selected to facilitate the clinicians interpretation, never to supersede it.

Only the software package facilities of SURVEY ANALYSIS will be considered. The package corresponds readily to data captured using the medical questionnaire, although it was originally designed for opinion polls, market research, traffic and other surveys. It accepts data in the previously described data representations, as alphanumeric variables, as binary variables, or as a number of soft data descriptors usually assigned as a series of numeric codes. It does expect to find complete data sets for each facet to be recorded and deficiencies in this area are overcome by use of designated data codes, or creating the catagories 'not known' and 'not recorded'.

The fundamental facility offered by this package is coordination. All the facets within a trial may be coordinated with all other facets to present a single overall representation of the required information. The same variable or group of variables may be examined and identical values or groups of values may be combined to produce distribution patterns showing the frequency with which they occur relative to the frequency of occurrence of other groups of variables (Table 13.1).

Output of the package is usually presented in the form of tables. Simple arithmetic means and standard errors may be calculated and included as part of the output (Table 13.2).

In practice the first stage in the use of both packages is the creation of a 'dictionary' of terms. This is normally done when the record design has been finalised. It consists of describing every facet which appears in the record and applies equally to the administrative data in the record as to the medical data. For example, age would be described as a two-digit field, which must always be present. If the trial is restricted to patients between 40 and 65 years old, then this would also be set in the dictionary limits. Any record presented to the package without an age record of between 40 and 65 would be rejected. The creation of the dictionary is a rather tedious, time consuming, but essential aspect of package usage.

The patient record forms are completed and the data converted via the key punch operator into a machine processable patient record. This record is read into the system and the content of the record is validated in keeping with the dictionary description. Errors are rejected, amended and represented to the system and the clinical trial data base is available for evaluation.

In practice we do not wait for the completion of the trial to commence the data evaluation. On receipt of 20 to 30 entry records, visit records and laboratory data recor

Table 13.1  Data coordinated at four levels

### ATROMID SURVEY ON LIPOPROTEIN LEVELS, ISRAEL (DR A HART)

RETINOPATHY

| | M 250 MG% | | | | M 250 MG% | | | | |
| | TREATED | | UNTREATED | | TREATED | | UNTREATED | | TOTAL |
| | MALE | FEMALE | MALE | FEMALE | MALE | FEMALE | MALE | FEMALE | |
|---|---|---|---|---|---|---|---|---|---|
| NR | 3 | 2 | 12 | 10 | 0 | 2 | 1 | 2 | 32 |
| NO | 51 | 56 | 46 | 46 | 28 | 25 | 30 | 23 | 305 |
| MODERATE | 1 | 1 | 2 | 3 | 1 | 2 | 0 | 1 | 11 |
| SEVERE | 0 | 0 | 1 | 0 | 0 | 0 | 0 | 0 | 1 |
| TOTAL | 55 | 59 | 61 | 59 | 29 | 29 | 31 | 26 | 349 |

Table 13.2 Standard errors and standard deviations using SURVEY ANALYSIS package

DR A BARNES DIABETIC SURVEY - TABLE OF STANDARD ERROR OF READINGS

|  | MALE | | FEMALE | |
|---|---|---|---|---|
|  | DIABETIC | CONTROL | DIABETIC | CONTROL |
| AGE | 2.23 | 1.47 | 2.12 | 1.60 |
| GLUCOSE | 19.36 | 2.20 | 22.05 | 1.68 |
| FIBRINOGEN | 24.37 | 14.74 | 24.59 | 13.42 |
| HAEMATOCRIT | 0.75 | 0.61 | 0.70 | 0.52 |
| V @ 0.77 | 1.39 | 0.57 | 1.38 | 0.86 |
| V @ 2.62 | 0.60 | 0.24 | 0.44 | 2.11 |
| V @ 23 | 0.14 | 0.12 | 0.15 | 0.12 |
| V @ 230 | 0.06 | 0.05 | 0.08 | 0.06 |

the information is punched and read into the system. This allows the system itself to be evaluated against 'real' data and pilot questions to be formulated by the clinician. Also at this stage we would prepare distribution counts which consist simply of all facets classified against the four main patient descriptors, male, female, drug, placebo (Table 13.3). This enables us to monitor at entry for balance between the drug and placebo group for all aspects of a trial. Where inbalance occurs this may be remedied by appropriate modification of the random allocation scheme.

As the trial progresses, questions evolve which allow best use of the system by creating question structures, whereby the same parameters may be used economically with a variety of data subsets (Table 13.4).

Using again as an example the intermittent claudication trial, the following pertiment data subsets; claudication site, progress since started treatment, femoral, popliteal, anterior and posterior tibial pulses, rest pain, vascular operation, ulcers, and onset of gangrene would be presented to the system and tables would be prepared corresponding to the question framework. SURVEY ANALYSIS is the major facility for the handling of all the clinical trial data.

The second data handling package, FIND-2, is used mostly in a complementary role. Although the package possesses a high degree of versatility, it is used primarily within our procedures to locate subgroups of patients or to reset data for subsequent analysis. Using the FIND-2 multiple enquiry system it is possible to ask a question involving a large number of facets, and each facet may be categorised on an 'and/or/ not/equals/not equals/between/ $>$/$<$/$\leq$/$\geq$' system of logic. In using this facility we have not found, as yet, any question which remotely approaches the full capacity of the package. The type of question that this facility answers is:

'Find how many (or which) patients are female, aged between 50 and 55, with a blood pressure greater than 90/110 at entry, suffering from diabetes, with a history of angina of effort, have had their cholesterol value lowered by a minimum of 20 units during the first six months of trial, and separate groups according to drug or placebo treatment'.

Table 13.3  Standard distribution counts covering male/female and drug/placebo

PRACTOLOL INTENSIVE CARE

PATIENTS WITHOUT CT (24 MONTH FOLLOW-UP)

INIT VHR  101

DISTRIBUTION OF PATIENTS BY WORK STATUS

|  | DRUG | | PLACEBO | | |
|  | MALE | FEMALE | MALE | FEMALE | TOTAL |
|---|---|---|---|---|---|
| NR | 4 | 1 | 9 | 4 | 18 |
| UNFIT FOR WORK | 4 | 6 | 6 | 1 | 17 |
| FIT FOR WORK | 2 | 1 | 2 | 0 | 5 |
| RES. OLD JOB | 12 | 2 | 15 | 1 | 30 |
| RES. LIGHT JOB | 4 | 1 | 4 | 0 | 9 |
| ACTIVE H'WIFE | 0 | 9 | 0 | 11 | 20 |
| ACTIVE RETIRED | 5 | 4 | 7 | 1 | 17 |
| TOTAL | 31 | 24 | 44 | 17 | 116 |

Table 13.4  Structured question format

|  |  | Drug Group | | Placebo Group | |
|  |  | Males | Females | Males | Females |
|---|---|---|---|---|---|
| Right side | 00 months 06 months 12 months 18 months |  |  |  |  |
| Left side | 00 months 06 months 12 months 18 months |  |  |  |  |

Although there is only a small amount of overlap between the two packages, many of the questions are such that they could be asked of either system. With some questions there is no difficulty in deciding which package to use. Questions like the one above and also simple questions such as 'How many people have attended the clinic for their 27 month visit?' would usually be done using the FIND-2 package. SURVEY ANALYSIS would be used for a related series of complex tabulations. For questions in the middle area, the decision to select a particular package is usually made on an arbitrary basis. This may depend on the preference of the individual doing the work or associated work being done on one of the packages.

There are problems with the system. Setting up the trial dictionaries and also setting up the more complex SURVEY ANALYSIS tabulations are tedious and time consuming. The fact that each trial creates a separate data base presents difficulties; for example, in bringing together all side effect data relating to a specific drug, or calculating how many patient months of therapy have been achieved. A further difficulty is that these are ICL packages and are not readily compatible with other non-ICL software. They are also machine orientated and can only be used on ICL installations. The latter problem can be overcome in some instances by the interchange of reformatted tapes. At worst, data from our system can always be recreated in punched card format.

The other two problems are prominent in our development area. Along with ICL we are evaluating a disc based prerelease version of SURVEY ANALYSIS which permits the use of more generalised instructions, reducing time required to specify complex questions. Independently, we are investigating the possibility of developing a front end onto the system which will permit us, at input, interrogation and retrieval to consider any specified series of trials as if it were only one.

We have now been using these two software packages for six years. We are satisfied with their wide applicability and capability. There are no problems with program amendments, enhancements or other maintenance. We see no reason why they will not continue to support our clinical trial procedure for the foreseeable future.

REFERENCES

British Medical Journal (1971) Trial of clofibrate in the treatment of ischaemic heart disease: five-year study by a group of physicians of the Newcastle upon Tyne region. *British Medical Journal,* **4**, 767 - 775.

British Medical Journal (1971) Ischaemic heart disease: a secondary prevention trial using clofibrate. Report by a research committee of the Scottish Society of Physicians. *British Medical Journal,* **4**, 775 - 784.

# 14.  Statistical Analysis of Trial Results

J. J. GRIMSHAW

Seven years have elapsed since the last AMAPI symposium on the Principles and Practice of Clinical Trials. It seems appropriate to look at some of the thoughts expressed on statistical analysis at that time (Grimshaw, 1970) and see what further problems may have emerged. It is apparent that scales of measurement and the combination of multicentre trial results are still the major problem areas: but let us take the 1969 issues in order and see where we stand today.

## Trial design

The sub-title of this chapter should be '... and the Interpretation Thereof' for one of the most important roles of the statistician is to interpret his numerical analysis in understandable terms. It is to focus on this aspect of his work that statistics are split between trials design and trials analysis in this book. It is easy to gain the impression that two entirely separate statistical exercises occur: first trial planning and then, after a long period, the trial analysis: In between is a long vacuum during which the statistician retires inside his black box.

This does not happen in practice because the completed trial never turns out as it was planned. Invariably some patients are lost to contact, patients are admitted outside the agreed entrance criteria, record sheets are mislaid (particularly those completed by patients themselves) and some laboratory studies are omitted or not recorded. However well designed the trial, we never finish with all the data we anticipated and even though in the design the statistician may have had a good idea of how he would like to handle the results, he never can do so in practice.

Table 14.1 illustrates a typical crossover design in two groups of patients. The appropriate analysis in this situation is a within patient comparison of drugs so that if one had 20 patients in each group, one would finish up with a comparison based on 40 differences. The purpose of the placebo periods is twofold: firstly to provide an independent measure of drug effect (for example, in Group 1 the best estimate of the response to drug A is obtained by comparing the response of a patient to drug A with his mean response to Placebo 1 and Placebo 2); and secondly to provide a washout period between active drugs.

But all too often on analysis the responses run Placebo 3>Placebo 2>Placebo 1 in both groups of patients. This may be an indication of gradual patient recovery or it could be an indication of carry over from the active drug into the placebo period. Although this gives us useful information about the duration of effect produced by the first administered drug, it does also suggest that the response to the second drug in

Table 14.1 A crossover design in two groups of patients

| |
| --- |
| Group 1: Placebo 1 - Drug A - Placebo 2 - Drug B - Placebo 3 |
| Group 2: Placebo 1 - Drug B - Placebo 2 - Drug A - Placebo 3 |

each case many be biased. Under these circumstances the only valid analysis may be to compare the effects produced by the first administered drugs *between* the two groups of patients, and then to estimate the total effects produced by administering the two drugs in the order A + B or B + A. Thus, final analysis depends very much on the trial design but even more strongly on how the trial was actually performed.

Perhaps the most important contribution of the statistician during the trial is to attempt to minimize the effects of deviations from the protocol. He can do this by modifying his ideas on final analytical procedures or, in cases of gross deviations from protocol, by modifying the design of the remainder of the trial.

### Editing and collating

There is little more to be said on this topic except to emphasize that it is probably the single most important aspect of clinical trial analysis. With the increasing trend towards trial complexity and record card design it is becoming more necessary for the statistician and medical adviser, or clinical trials assistant, to take a joint look at the edited data before analysis is started.

As shown in chapters 6 and 13, data collection, transmission, compilation and analysis are increasingly becoming automated. However, editing is still mostly a manual task. We can programme the computer to flag input values outside designated normal ranges and to perform similar rote rasks. But editing also involves the ability to observe a pattern in the results collected from one investigator; for example, suggesting a particular type of doctor patient relationship, or a bias in recording some of the data, or even a set of fraudulent entries. Such tasks can only be manually performed and make editing the rate determining factor in the production of the final clinical trial report.

### Scales of measurement

Quantitative variables, such as blood pressure and haemoglobin concentration, present little difficulty either in collection or subsequent analysis. A range of powerful statistical tests can be applied from 't' tests and ANOVA for between group comparisons to regression analysis for between group association. The problems arise when we look at variables which are really qualitative but which we would like to handle as numerically as possible. Let us consider a typical example of such a variable, the assessment of pain.

Leaving aside the several quantitative methods of assessing experimental pain, in a clinical situation pain is usually recorded in one of three different ways:

We can ask the patient to record the change in pain after treatment.

We can ask patients to assess the degree of pain on each occasion. If we verbalise his responses we can construct scales such as are shown in Table 14.2.

Instead of using verbal scales we can ask the patient to mark a visual analogue scale.

Table 14.2  Two alternative methods for assessment of pain relief

| Comparison with pre-treatment | | Degree of pain (measured on two or more occasions) | |
| --- | --- | --- | --- |
| Category | Score | Category | Score |
| Cured | 3 | Absent | 0 |
| Much Improved | 2 | Mild | 1 |
| Some Improvement | 1 | Moderate | 2 |
| No Change | 0 | Severe | 3 |
| Worse | -1 | Very Severe | 4 |
| Much Worse | -2 | | |

Let us leave method 3 for the time being and concentrate on the first two ways which are equivalent in terms of the following discussion. For each of these systems of response we have devised a series of categories that form an ordinal scale, that is in the order written, each category is 'worse' than the one preceding it in an understandable way. On such data we can play the numbers game. That is, we can compare two drugs either as a crossover within patients, or between two groups of patients depending on circumstances, by comparing frequencies in each category by the appropriate $x^2$ test. If numbers in the cells are small we can combine adjacent frequencies; that is a perfectly admissible operation for ordinal data.

To test the significance of a single drug effect we can perform $x^2$ tests between the combined group 'cured and much improved' and 'much worse' and also between 'some improvement' and 'worse'. If numbers are small it is better to collapse the data into the two groups 'improved' and 'worse' and test the significance of a single drug effect by a Sign Test (Siegel, 1956). With very small numbers we can use the powerful Fisher Exact Test. These are purely qualitative ways of handling the data but the disadvantage of $x^2$ is that it is associated with large Type II errors, it is easy to miss a real difference between products.

The first way of attempting to 'strengthen' the data is to apply a numerical scale to each category and, *in the absence of any good clinical reason to the contrary,* probably the best one can do is to apply linear scales such as are shown in Table 14.2. There are strong objections to considering such data to be normally distributed although Fisher has proposed the use of a normalising transformation of ordinal scores. However, the distribution free equivalents to the 't' tests are the Wilcoxon Signed Ranks Test and the Mann Whitney Test for paired and unpaired data respectively. These very powerful alternatives are strongly recommended in such situations.

There are two problems in applying such tests: Firstly with restricted scales, such as these, there are always a large number of 'ties' in the data which weaken the tests considerably; Secondly, the moment one begins to aggregate scores, either across patients or between different assessments on the same patient, the exact linearity of the scale is an important assumption, that is we are saying not only that $4 > 3 > 2$ but that $4 - 3 = 3 - 2$. This is equivalent to saying that pain is a continuum and we are asking patients to discriminate equal quanta within the continuum. This does not seem too unreasonable an assumption.

But if patients can distinguish equal increments of pain, could we not derive a more informative scale which, at the same time, would get rid of ties? This leads into a consideration of the third method of recording pain response, the use of visual analogue scales.

The patient is asked to imagine pain stretching from 'none' to 'as severe as it could be' and to mark the scale correspondingly. This method has been used by many workers (Aitken, 1969). In theory, it removes the constriction placed on the patient by employing a limited range of semantic differentials. Huskisson (1974) has looked at some of the problems in applying the technique to assessment of pain and, in an interesting experiment, used a scale with the guide words 'severe', 'moderate' and 'mild' superimposed. He found, perhaps predictably, that 73 per cent of the patients 'homed-in' on one of the guide words and did not take advantage of the additional sensitivity of the scale.

Even if one assumed that patients can distinguish up to 20 grades of pain (equivalent to measuring a distance on a 10 cm line to the nearest 0.5 cm) the gain may be illusory. At some stage one is faced with the problem of aggregating across patients and this implies that one patient's 3.5 cm is equivalent to another's. This seems rather more unlikely than implying that two ratings of 'moderate pain' are equivalent to each other. It is not at all certain that relying on semantic differentials is any less meaningful than applying an arbitrary numerical scale.

To summarize, we are dealing with an area where a response can be verbalised or, with some reservations, semiquantified or even quantified. In either case one is faced with the problems of aggregation. It could well be that, in the long run, the most robust procedure is to divide the data into 'improved' and 'worse'. Unless one has considerable experience in handling such data more sophisticated methods such as visual analogue scales are probably best avoided.

### Aggregation of symptom scores

We may wish to aggregate symptom scores for two reasons:

1. In a trial in which several readings of one parameter are recorded it may be of interest to derive a patient's total, or average, response over a period.

2. Where several parameters are recorded for the same patient we may wish to arrive at some overall global view of the patient's condition.

The first case is relatively straight forward *providing* there is no evidence of a trend over time. For example in hypertensive trials it is quite common for a patient to be titrated to a maximum tolerated dose and then assessed at monthly intervals for, say, six months. The first thing to do is to examine the last six months' data and ensure that there has been neither a steady trend during the period nor a sudden dramatic change to a new value. Either effect could possibly indicate the development of dependence, for example. In cases of doubt regression analysis or similar techniques can be used to show the absence of a significant time dependent effect. It is then quite reasonable to reduce 'within patient' variation by averaging, say, the last three months' figures. If a trend over the six months exists it is still numerically possible to average over the six months to arrive at a total response over the period but it is obvious that this is not a meaningful figure. The appropriate analysis in such cases is to assess drug effects at varying intervals of time and gain the maximum possible in information from the trial.

The situation where we wish to aggregate several symptoms in the same patient is more complex. A typical area where this occurs is the assessment of rheumatoid arthritis. Let us consider just three of the possible measures one might make: pain at night, severity of morning stiffness and pain during the day. Not forgetting the earlier discussion let us assume for the moment that each is assessed by the patient on a four point scale and that each parameter has been summed over 14 days. Typical responses that one might obtain are shown in Table 14.3.

Table 14.3  Individual assessment scores and the global estimate

| Patient | Night Pain | Morning Stiffness | Day Pain | Total Score? |
|---------|-----------|-------------------|----------|--------------|
| 1 | 36 | 24 | 34 | 94 |
| 2 | 30 | 28 | 36 | 94 |

Inspection of the individual parameters reveals that patient number one had a 20 per cent higher night pain score than patient two, a 14 per cent lower score for morning stiffness and much the same day pain score. The question is: Are we gaining any more information by saying the total score is the same for each patient? It may well be that in making valid comparisons between drugs it is the distribution of scores that is more meaningful than the total response.

Even if one does wish to aggregate numerical scores in some way, simple linear addition may not be the best procedure. The only theoretically acceptable way of combining scores is to perform a principal component analysis and to work on the first two or three components. Even then, the stability of these components has to be checked between two or more drugs and between two or more assessment points depending on the trial design. This procedure is becoming easier, with the availability of computer packages which simplify the matrix algebra involved. It sometimes happens that a study of the two or three major components identifies sub groups within a syndrome or yields other clinically useful information.

The simplest way of handling multiple symptom data is to set up success/fail criteria for each symptom in turn, on acceptable clinical grounds. If one allows a third category of 'no change' it is possible to set up acceptance rules such as:

All symptoms improve = success.

Some symptoms unchanged, the rest improved, none worse = partial success.

Any symptoms worse = failure.

Since the presence of clinically significant side effects or any drug induced reason for withdrawal can be handled in the same overall assessment it is clear that this provides a quick, powerful, global estimate which can be analysed by the methods discussed earlier. In my opinion it is unlikely that any clinically meaningful difference will be missed by such a procedure providing the trial has been otherwise properly controlled and monitored.

### Demographic factors and general practice trials

General practice trials have received much adverse publicity over the past months. Some authorities have seemed to suggest that the only 'acceptable' clinical trials are those performed in selected hospitals prior to marketing. Yet reliance on within hospital trials, however well performed they may have been, can be very misleading. The first reason for this is that patients referred to hospital are often the more severely affected with a particular disease or those with a long standing condition refractory to several alternative treatments. In such cases it is by no means necessarily true that success or failure in hospitalised patients implies a corresponding response in general practice patients.

The second problem in attempting to extrapolate to a wider population is the fantastic 'mix' that comprises the UK population. Age, sex, occupation, ethnic group, environmental influences and other such factors vary enormously from practice to practice. In order to predict what drug effectiveness will be, as prescribed, it is essential at some stage in the product marketing phase to perform a multipractice trial covering as wide a patient mix as possible.

The drawbacks to such a demographic addition to trials data are first that it is sometimes difficult to assess such factors (how does one record the socioeconomic group of a housewife?); second, that it may prove an expensive exercise. To fully analyse multiple demographic data we require hundred of patients rather than tens and conceivably, thousands rather than hundreds. We have to be prepared at the statistical analysis stage to sort out some of these factors if we are really going to understand how our new drug is acting.

### Scientific or marketing trials

Closely related to the last topic is the different approach to trials which can be termed scientific medicine (Phase II) and those which are more marketing oriented (Phases III and IV). Sometimes the differences are small, although the topic can generate a good deal of argument. It is naive to imagine either that a 'scientific' trial has no marketing potential or that it is possible to perform a useful 'marketing' trial that does not seek to answer a specific medical question. There is, however, an important difference in the statistical handling of such trials. Put simply it is the difference between estimation and prediction.

At the stage in new drug development when a drug first passes into clinical pharmacology we are doing little more than establishing the drug's bioavailability in the human animal. The licensing authorities rightly demand an increasingly sophisticated pathology back up when the drug is first prescribed to patients. The first clinical trials performed are *intensive*, on comparatively few patients but generating vast quantities of medical and scientific data. If one is seeking to establish the scientific basis for a difference between drugs such trials are ideal. At the analysis stage we perform ANOVA and similar procedures to identify and remove from the comparison any extraneous influences that we have not been able to control. In this way we obtain the maximum possible precision in the estimation of medical and scientific differences between drugs or different preparations of the same drug.

The dilemma lies in the fact that as one increases scientific discrimination by such control procedures one necessarily obtains a weaker prediction of the total performance of the drug when launched. To overcome this we perform trials on a marketed product on an *extensive* basis, relying on large numbers of patients and the Central Limit Theorem to provide the best overall estimate of potential drug performance. In the analysis of such trials, although we may be interested in a comparison between drugs, we tend not to remove the extraneous variables for now we are interested in a prediction of what sort of differences will be seen in practice. If we can identify the nuisance variables the more meaningful technique is to build up a multivariable regression equation so that we can predict response under a wide variety of conditions.

These conflicting aims at different stages of the product's life do not always seem to be fully understood by the licensing authorities.

**Conflicting data from multicentre trials**

Assuming that, for the reasons already outlined, a multicentre trial is performed, what do we do when two separate centres yield different, perhaps diametrically opposite, conclusions? This is a contentious area and is worth examining in some detail.

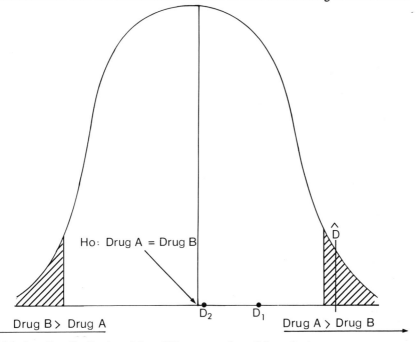

Fig. 14.1 Sampling distribution of drug difference on the null hypothesis
   Hatched areas are rejection regions for Ho: A = B at $P < 0.5$
   $\hat{D}$ = observed difference between drugs
   $D_1$ $D_2$ = two alternative values for true difference between drugs

Figure 14.1 illustrates the sampling distribution of the difference between two drugs A and B on the null hypothesis, Ho: A=B. The two rejection regions are equivalent to accepting the alternative hypothesis, $H_1$: A $\neq$ B, with drug A better than drug B and drug B better than drug A respectively. In Figure 14.1 an observed difference, $\hat{D}$ is shown as coming just inside the conventional 5 per cent rejection region and we would conclude from this trial that drug A was superior.

However, the true difference is unknown. In the figure it is shown in two alternative positions, $D_1$ and $D_2$ and for each of these cases we can imagine a prior distribution of mean drug difference centred at $D_1$ and $D_2$ respectively. It can be seen that if the true drug difference is $D_1$, $\hat{D}$ is a likely outcome and repeated drug trials will yield an overall drug difference tending towards $D_1$ with a final mean not so very different from $\hat{D}$. On the other hand, if the true drug difference is $D_2$, the observed difference $\hat{D}$ is not quite so likely but by no means an impossible outcome: It would certainly occur more often than once in 20 trials on average. Now if we perform repeated trials we will tend to an overall mean value approaching $D_2$. The final mean will not be close to $\hat{D}$ and, furthermore, we will quite often obtain results indicating that B is the better drug. Occasionally we may find a result so extreme that it occurs in the other rejection region for the null hypothesis and we will say drug B is 'significantly better' than drug A. It is evident that the smaller the true drug difference is the more likely we are to obtain conflicting results in repeated trials. Furthermore these differing results have nothing to do with the way in which the trial has been conducted or reported.

We are moving towards the situation where for many diseases available therapy is so effective that any improvement can only, at best, be marginal, for example a ten day course of penicillin for gram negative urinary tract infections. In such circumstances two things become apparent: We can *expect* conflicting results between trials; and we are going to require a very large number of results before we can establish whether a difference does, in fact, exist.

Superimposed on these problems are the 'between practice' differences discussed in the last section. There we saw how a consistent drug effect could produce inconsistent results due to a different patient mix between practices. In this section we have seen how even with 'consistent' patients one can still obtain conflicting results if the drug difference is small.

Multicentre trials have the dual purpose of balancing out between practice differences and at the same time producing an overall estimate of true drug effect. However, their interpretation places one in what may be called a moral dilemma. It is good statistical practice to average out the results of several contemporary trials in order to obtain the best mean estimate of drug effect. But how should one publish such results?

The only valid procedure would seem to be to publish all the data in one statement containing a single estimate of the mean response together with an indication of the expected range. Unfortunately there are two sources of pressure which may be brought to bear upon medical advisers in an attempt to secure selective publication. First, marketing departments are, somewhat naturally, keen to have publications showing their product in the best light; after all this provides the most cogent representative 'detail'. Secondly, and perhaps more laudably, individual centres may wish to see their own input published as an independent feature. This is particularly true where international trials are concerned.

As we have seen, the smaller the true between drug difference the more likely we are to obtain conflicting results. Failure to understand this basic fact has led to widespread misinterpretation of trial results. Perhaps in areas where we are close to producing the ideal drug the only option available to us in the future will be to insist on a single, definitive all embracing publication.

REFERENCES

Aitken, R.C.B. (1969) A growing edge of measurement of feelings, *Proc. Roy. Soc. Med.* **62**, 989.
Grimshaw, J.J. (1970) Statistical analysis of clinical trial results. In *The Principles and Practice of Clinical Trials,* pages 112 - 125, E.& S. Livingstone.
Huskisson, E.C. (1974) Measurement of pain, *Lancet,* 1127.
Siegal, S. (1956) *Non-parametric Statistics for the Behavioral Sciences,* McGraw Hill Book Company Inc.

# 15. Presentation of Results

C. F. HAWKINS

Writing in journals and speaking at meetings are the usual means of presenting results of research. However, the first step is to give a talk either at a seminar or before a group of colleagues. This audience provides an opportunity for criticism so that faults can be detected at an early stage.

## Writing in journals

Original articles usually consist of about 2,000 words, short reports 600 and letters not more than 400 words. A high percentage of articles are rejected by editors or their referees. This happens for the following reasons: they are too long; nothing original is reported; the logic or validity of results is doubtful; or they are written badly.

Thinking must be done before starting to write, else time is wasted. All facts, ideas, and references to previous work should be assembled and then a detailed plan prepared. The first draft can be written or dictated, but beware the tape recorder for it encourages verbosity. The first draft should be typed roughly in double spacing with wide margins and a 'blue pencil' used ruthlessly. Several editions may be necessary before the final draft. Somerset Maugham revised his manuscript six times; hence the clarity of his writing.

The writer should decide upon the journal to which the article will be submitted and study the layout and style of papers already published in it. Most journals include 'Notes for Contributors' or 'Suggestions to Authors' and these should be the guide (Brit. med. J., 1976). The conventional outline of an article is: 1. *Title.* This deserves careful thought as the title first catches the reader's eye. It will be included in Index Medicus, so do consider the person who has to index it. Make it short though sufficiently descriptive, without one unnecessary word and no abbreviations. 2. *Introduction.* A good beginning should tempt readers to read on and be intelligible to ordinary readers however specialised the subject. 3. *Material (or patients) and methods.* Here is described means by which investigations were carried out. Enough detail must be given to allow repetition of methods. 4. *Results.* Just give the results succinctly. These should be facts and not comments, which should be put in the discussion. A normal range of values should be mentioned when necessary. Tables and figures are used but the data should not be in the text as well. 5. *Discussion.* The significance of results is discussed and conclusions given. Recapitulation of results should be avoided. 6. *Summary.* The summary is the article's most important part. Many will only read the summary and it may be reproduced throughout the world. It should be brief and clear with just the essential points. It must not be a rehash of the article and no new facts must be mentioned.

It should be informative and not merely descriptive. An example of the two types was given by the editor of the Lancet (1937):

*Descriptive type:* A series of cases of food poisoning is reported and their causation discussed.

*Informative or factual type:* Fifteen people fell ill with vomiting an hour after eating lizard soup. Skin tests showed that they were hypersensitive to lizards.

7. *Acknowledgements.* A list should be made in order to avoid forgetting anyone. Those mentioned should include everyone without whose special help the article could not have been written. Those who have carried out routine investigations like radiography or blood tests need not be included unless something special has been done. Research bodies who have given grants or pharmaceutical firms who have sponsored the study or provided the drug must be mentioned. Be simple without effusiveness.

8. *References.* Collect these properly at the start, preferably on index cards, else time will be wasted chasing up lost references when the article is ready. Never include articles not seen or read. A current issue of the journal should be consulted to find out about the format; for example, whether to include titles and references in full or abbreviated and also to find out details of punctuation and if first and last page numbers are demanded. The Harvard system whereby authors names and date are given in the text and references at the end of the paper in alphabetical order is commonly used. All names are given when the reference is first quoted; '*et al.*' or 'and others' when there are more than two authors, when referred to afterwards. The alternative method is to give numbers only in the text. If there is doubt as to how to quote a reference, perhaps in an obscure journal, it should be written out completely.

### The manuscript

The article should be typed on A4 paper on one side only with pages numbered consecutively. Double spaced typing must be used with generous margins (at least 4 cm at top, bottom and left, and 2.5 cm at right) to leave room for editor's corrections. Good paper should be used. Double spacing is necessary throughout for separate title page, legends of illustrations, foot notes and references.

Illustrations and tables should be put on separate sheets. A soft pencil, at least 2B, should be used to write on the back of the print as follows: the word TOP, the author's name in the middle, and the figure number at the bottom. A print can be damaged by a hard pencil or paper clip. Legends for illustration should be typed on a separate sheet. Before the final draft is typed, go over the rough draft with the current issue of the journal at hand and study every detail. For example, check the layout of the title page with the author's name (usually initials for men though full christian name is allowed for women), and note whether degrees are needed and so on. Points especially to check are: consistency in typing per cent or %, or spelling out numbers up to 10 and otherwise typing as figures, the use of capitals and abbreviations (always give complete word or term in full when first used and with abbreviation after it), consistency in symbols (some journals like 15 mg. and others 15 mg), names of drugs (patented products including proprietary drugs should begin with a capital but otherwise written with small letters). Footnotes should be avoided as far as possible for they interrupt the reader and are expensive; but if these are necessary they should be typed on separate sheets and numbered consecutively with the article. The top copy should always be left with the typist and only copies altered or shown to co-authors; the typist herself will then deal with any corrections and the top copy will not be spoiled. This should be sent to the editor with any copies as requested by the journal. Pages should be fixed together with paper clips and not pins or staples, for the compositor has to type each sheet separately. One should make sure that it is packed properly when posted and cardboard used to protect prints. The name and address of the person to whom proofs are to be sent should be included. 'Good copy' is the printer's description of a perfect manuscript easy to handle.

To get a paper published quickly, it should be easily understood by both editor and reader without the need to ponder over it. It should appear exactly in every way as other articles in the journal. The editor may accept it completely or perhaps suggest resubmission when revised or shortened. If rejected, it could be sent to another journal or rewritten as a short communication for one which encourages these, or as a letter. Letters with new or unusual facts are indexed in the Index Medicus.

### Faults in writing

A good style for writing can be defined as the maximum amount of information in the minimum number of words, written in a pleasing way. Unfortunately there are many doctors and scientists who, although able to think and speak clearly, cannot transmit their thoughts in writing. This is one reason why threequarters of the articles submitted to some journals are rejected. Scientific writing must be so clear that it can easily be understood in Russia or China as well as in America and Britain. The most serious fault is when simple matters are made to appear unintelligible because of long windedness, or when polysyllabic words or pseudo-scientific profundity are used. This muddled style of writing has been called barnacular by Ivor Brown in England and gobbledygook by Maury Maverick in the USA; the editor of *Lancet* described it as 'the pompous circumlocution often imagined appropriate to scientific publication'. Verbosity is illustrated by the following:

| *Several words instead of one* | |
| --- | --- |
| A considerable amount of | much |
| A decreased amount of | less |
| An increased amount of | more |
| Present in association with | accompany |
| Cells of the monuclear type | mononuclears |
| Come to the same conclusion | agree |
| Decreased in weight | lighter |
| Due to the fact that | because |
| Encountered more frequently | commoner |
| Has been engaged in a study of | has studied |
| Not in accordance with the facts | false |
| Present only in small numbers | scanty |
| Presents a picture similar to | resembles |
| There can be little doubt that this is | this is probably |
| *Long-winded phrases* | |
| An upper intestinal barium study | Barium meal |
| Roentgenographic study | X-ray |

| On an out-patient basis | As an out-patient |
|---|---|
| Assume the recumbent position | Lie down |

*Superfluous statements.* Unnecessary qualifying words are another source of verbiage. Authors should, whenever possible, take responsibility rather than hiding behind such terms as:

Authorities agree that...

It is recognised that...

It is a well known fact that...

Similarly, vague introductory statements may kill whole sentences. The following are typical cliches:

Although certainly not a new finding, it is important to point out that...

A difference of opinion exists regarding...

I have no hesitation in saying...

It has been proposed that...

It is interesting to note that...

It is the purpose of this paper...

It should be emphasized that...

Sentences should be short. Readers need the pause of a full stop to think and are confused by long passages without interruption. Sentences of twenty words or less are best, for they are easier to read and write. Short sentences are also the choice of great writers, especially when describing events of action or history, and convey the impression of speed as well as aiding in rapid understanding. In contrast, a long sentence gives an air of solemnity and deliberation to writing, so that even a trivial subject can be given grandeur and dignity, and be endowed with fictitious seriousness.

The active rather than passive tense should be used, for words are then saved and writing becomes more vigorous:

| It is possible that the cause | The cause may be |
|---|---|
| The incision was made by him | He made the incision |
| It was reported by Smith | Smith reported |

Clarity of writing can be easily assessed by reading it aloud, either alone or to a critic, perhaps one's wife. Tongue twisters are detected and punctuation checked, for when the voice needs a pause, the text requires a stop.

## Speaking at meetings

Speaking is an art by itself. The temptation to use an article, perhaps already in the press, as the text for a talk should be resisted. It is better to plan the communication anew. Speech should be looser in texture, and less detailed than writing. The listener must accept the speed chosen by the speaker, whereas the reader can select his own pace, lingering over difficult passages or skipping quickly over pieces of less interest and importance. When listening, continuous attention is needed; there is no time to pause or to study an illustration again. One unknown word which makes the listener stumble, stop, and think, may cause loss of contact with the speaker. So the speaker must speak clearly and simply, indicating when he is moving on to the next point, for the listener does not have ideas separated by punctuation or paragraphs, or perhaps repeat key points. No one wants to hear a speaker 'talking like a book'.

Some speakers have a natural ability to make an interesting subject dull or a simple one complicated; others can imbue a complicated subject with an interest and clarity which captivates their audience. The fact is that the clearer the delivery the harder the work that has to be put into the preparation. The person who boasts that he has put his talk together in the train on the way to the meeting may sometimes be brilliant; more often the listener may wish that the journey had been longer, or not undertaken at all.

## Form and style

The simple pattern 'beginning, middle, end' should be followed. A short introduction is a natural courtesy to those unfamiliar with the subject and there is seldom an audience so specialised as not to appreciate this. However, too long introductions can be irritating especially when repeating the same theme as in a conference concerning a single subject. The purpose of the talk is to bring out the three or more points that can be made in ten or fifteen minutes and not to report work that has been done over several years. Strict pruning of unnecessary or complex data is essential. Details, like tables, list of figures, and experimental methods can be available in a handout to anyone interested. Any fool can make things sound complicated; it is the clever man whose audience understands his talk. There is a story in one learned society that when young, inexperienced research workers come to give a talk, they are warned 'remember you are addressing a most distinguished assembly of scientists. Therefore you should speak to them as though they are children of four years of age'. Slight hyperbole perhaps, but it is a pity that more speakers do not follow this guide.

## Timing

A speaker who exceeds his allotted time without permission from the chairman may upset the entire plan of a meeting. Time may have to be stolen from other speakers or the discussion curtailed. The shorter the paper, the more popular the speaker. It is better to aim at one or two minutes less than the full time allowed. For it is difficult to estimate the time needed for showing slides and time spent drawing on the blackboard or overhead projector is notoriously unpredictable.

## Causes of obscurity

Sometimes the word 'communication' is a misnomer. 'Too many papers take the form of an inaudible soliloquy in front of a series of invisible tables', according to a member of the pathological society. Simplifying a technical subject is difficult. Speakers confuse, and so quickly lose the interest of, their audience for the following reasons:

*Too much detail.* The material may consist of work that has taken one or more years. Any attempt to cram all the data into a short communication will obscure the message.

*Inability to explain.* Communications are commonly given as if the listener were perfectly familiar with the speaker's special interest, for someone working intensively for a long time on a special problem often cannot imagine what it is like not to know all that he knows.

*Jargon.* As different branches of medicine develop each creates its own vocabulary which is understood only by those habitually using it. This private language or jargon is necessary for easy communication and saves much time. However, one of these words when unexplained may cause a listener to stop and ponder; and contact with the speaker may never be regained. Abbreviations without explanation are frustrating to those unfamiliar with them. Symbols such as CCF, BRR, IUGT and PPLO may be obvious to the reader but there may be some who stumble over them.

*Speaking too quickly.* It is particularly important to avoid this at international meetings when interpreters are doing their best to translate.

*Reading instead of speaking.* Most societies have a rule that communications must be spoken and not read. Reading, unless by an expert, is impersonal; and a paper read rapidly in a monotone becomes almost meaningless. The natural rhythm of telling a story, with its pauses and its contact with the audience, is lost. There are exceptions to this rule: international meetings when a speaker has to give a paper in another language; then the speaker should practise reading it intelligently beforehand. For the speaker who lacks confidence in speaking from notes, a compromise is possible. If the talk is first typed and practised again and again, the script gradually becomes unnecessary until only a few key phrases, suitably underlined, are needed. The result of this is either a memorised speech helped by key phrases, or an extemporary speech prompted and held together by manuscript. Most speakers use notes, usually on cards. These should be fixed together preferably by a ring in case they are accidently dropped.

### Incomprehensible slides

Just as the first requirement in a speaker is audibility, so the first test of a slide is legibility. Yet at nearly every meeting slides are shown that are unreadable unless the audience is equipped with field glasses. In the ten or fifteen seconds given to showing a slide, only three or four lines can be read. Yet the slides may be packed with ten or twenty lines of details which the reader has spent months in preparing. This overcrowded slide (Figure 15.1) often resembles a page from a railway timetable. It is a pity that photographers and those in departments of medical illustration cannot smother these at birth.

No slide should be shown unless it can be read by the back row of the audience. A simple way of insuring this is to make the lettering large enough to be read by the naked eye without projection. This also helps when sorting slides before a talk. Slides should be discussed first with the staff of the department of medical illustration, as much of their time can be wasted by requests for useless slides (Hawkins and Dee, 1973). All material should be scrutinized to find the best way of showing it pictorially, whether by graph, histogram or diagram. Statistical data, such as columns of figures and tables, can be converted into pictures showing relationships and trends, to illustrate the ideas derived from the data. The design of a slide should be simple and open with plenty of space and its meaning obvious without explanation. Generally, one idea only should be illustrated in each slide, lettering should be limited to about three or four lines, and graphs should contain no more than three or four curves. Tables should be kept to four

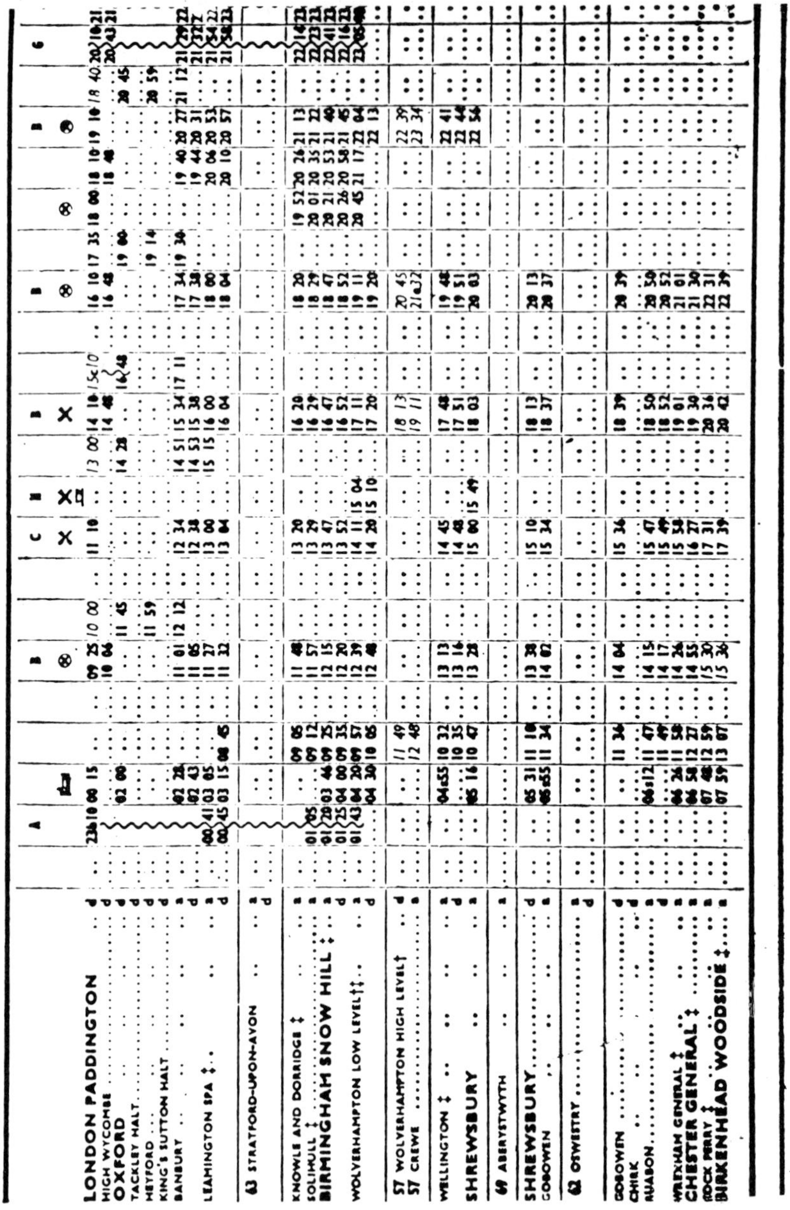

Fig. 15.1

columns and four horizontal lines, sixteen entries altogether. Important figures can be coloured or put in heavy print to draw the attention of the audience to them. Slides should be prepared well beforehand and every detail, especially statistics, checked with the same fastidious attention that is given to correcting proofs. Radiographs or photomicrographs should only be shown when there is sufficient contrast. An explanatory drawing in the corner of the radiograph or a marker on the photomicrograph will help those seeing it for the first time.

The perfect slide needs little or no explanation. Preferably it should be designed so that the speaker does not have to point or look at it except to check that the projectionist has not made a mistake. If there is reading matter, the speaker must keep silent and allow the audience to read it. This is a common error today. Speakers read the writing on a slide as if the listeners were halfwitted or unable to read. All that is needed is a period of silence and then the attention of the audience can be drawn to one or two points. Slides must be projected beforehand, for they may look different on the screen, a fact which accounts for the speaker who gazes at his slide in some perplexity trying to recognise it. The original typescript or drawing of a slide can be included in the speaker's notes to save him having to turn his back to the audience to look at the screen.

*Other visual aids*

The blackboard is a simple, flexible and inexpensive way of illustrating a talk, although its skillful use is often handicapped by poor illumination and a bad surface. It is easy to make simple mistakes: standing in front of what is written; continuing to talk while writing on the blackboard so that one's voice becomes inaudible; making the writing too small; starting to erase from below upwards before it has been read. However, blackboards or 'white boards' can only be used during seminars when reporting the work at a preliminary stage for there is insufficient time during formal meetings.

The overhead projector has the advantage that the speaker faces the audience and has eye contact with them. Transparencies (acetate sheets) can be prepared beforehand and much ingenuity can be used in preparing several overlays. Diagrams can be partly prepared and finished during the talk. There is also a fitment for slides so that an overhead projector can be used throughout the talk.

*The projectionist*

The speaker depends upon the projectionist who can ruin his talk through incompetence. However, he is apt to be taken for granted when all goes well. He must be given slides in correct order, each marked to indicate the correct way of insertion; the speaker's name should be marked on the box. Some speakers forget that there is a limit to the rate at which slides can be shown, and that projectionists being human may make mistakes. Incorrect focusing is a frustrating fault for fine slides may then be spoilt. It is seldom necessary for the lecture theatre to be blacked out, except for when showing coloured slides or X-rays. All that is usually needed is for the lights to be dimmed, then the speaker can see the audience to whom he is talking.

*Points to check before the meeting*

Technology, while improving efficiency, has made the modern lecture theatre more complex. In particular, the two actors, the lecturer and his projectionist, may be separated. Fortunately there is usually a two way microphone or telephone in the projectionist's compartment; otherwise the only way to communicate is by signal and this must be agreed upon before the lecture. The method of signalling about slides must be checked, either by buzzer or by speaking directly to the projectionist. The lectern should be studied, and most important is the light for glancing at notes when slides are being shown, so the site of the switch should be noted. Other points to check are the position of the rod or torch for pointing to the slides, the site of the chalk if the blackboard is going to be used, and the microphone.

## REFERENCES

British Medical Journal (1976) Instructions to authors. *British Medical Journal,* **1**, 6.
Hawkins, C.F. & Dee, T.F. (1973). The department of medical illustration: use and abuse. *Medical and Biological Illustration,* **23**, 74 - 77.
Lancet (1937) On writing for the Lancet. *Lancet,* **1**, 1.

## FURTHER READING

Asher, R. (1958) Why are medical articles so dull? *British Medical Journal,* **2**, 502.
Hawkins, C.F. (1967) *Speaking and Writing in Medicine: The Art of Communication.* Illinois USA, Charles C. Thomas.
O'Connor, M. & Woodford, F.P. (1975) Writing scientific papers in English.. Amsterdam and New York. *Excerpta Medica.*
Thorne, C. (1970) *Better Medical Writing.* London: Pitman.

# Discussion Part 3

*Dr. G. Beaumont (Geigy):* I agree with Dr. Galbraith about the question of enthusiasm. One of the biggest problems we have at the moment, is having agreed a protocol and generated the enthusiasm, maintaining the enthusiasm for several months whilst waiting to be granted a clinical trial certificate. It is a difficult problem for all of us at the moment.

*Dr. Galbraith:* There is no secret here. Continual visits from the coordinator are best, with possibly a dummy run of some part of the design. Recently an investigator was anxious to try using the visual analogue scale (VAS). This has drawbacks particularly amongst the elderly who have great difficulty in using it. I suggested that he run a pilot study of the VAS alone in clinical use. An idea like this can maintain enthusiasm and iron out some of the difficulties which otherwise may only appear during the actual trial itself.

*Chairman:* Dr. Marsh, you mention the cooperation of the trialist with ancillary staff. If he goes to all members of staff, they may also ask for payment. This would put up the total cost.

*Dr. Marsh:* I agree. It depends on the investigator and the situation. The trialist should go and see ancillary staff *only* with the agreement of the investigator. You must discuss with him the use of ancillary investigations and decide between yourselves whether other staff should be included.

*Dr. A.M. Edwards (Fisons):* I endorse what Dr. Marsh says about attention to detail paying dividends. Dr. Nicholson said that he thought a medical adviser could look after fifteen current trials. Would you agree with that figure or would you think that a smaller number is more practical?

*Dr. Marsh:* There is no set number. It depends on what type of trials you are looking after, how big they are and what they involve. If you had an enormous multicentre trial, it may take up all your time; but you could otherwise handle twenty or thirty small open studies.

*Dr. J. Domenet (Geigy):* I wish to reinforce a point Dr. Harcus made. A word of caution ought to be given about large surveillance studies such as the Boston group. These groups record everything that happens to everybody on every drug and then they do thousands of correlations and find something significant. This is hardly surprising, as by chance you will find something significant. I think they have a duty not to start a scare until they have done the prospective study which confirms their findings.

*Dr. Harcus:*  I would agree with that. All methods have their drawbacks and their advantages. We have to take the good points from each particular method and try to be aware of the bad points.

*Dr. B.T. Marsh (Leo):*  What if you find severe adverse reaction, such as a fetal abnormality? Are you going to do a prospective study or wait? You must consider what these groups report, but it must be related to the risk and the chances of finding out the exact cause.

*Dr. Harcus:*  We should take a more aggressive attitude in monitoring adverse reactions. Fetal abnormality is one way that we might do this. Eventually one of the drugs that we investigate will produce fetal abnormality. I encourage my staff to go out and record all normal deliveries, so that when an abnormality occurs, perhaps we can get some idea of the context.

*Dr. C. Kratochvil (Upjohn Europe):*  When an adverse reaction is reported, go out and look at the records personally. I have done this many times. I am appalled to find that many times the incriminated drug was never given. This happens too frequently. The status of hospital records and the quality of the data is appallingly bad in England. There is literally too much garbage in the literature and it is time we cleaned it up.

*Dr. T. Pulvertaft (Zyma):*  Dr. Harcus, how long do you leave a trial going on before you decide that it is dead? For example a trial has been going on for four years, you have 38 patients in it and the design called for 42. Each time you want to close the trial, the investigator says he must really finish it off, and will have another two patients next week. At what stage do you say 'no more'?

*Dr. Harcus:*  These are the trials that should be closed. These people are very nice when you go to see them. They promise you the earth but at the end of four years there is still nothing. It depends on how long each patient is studied. If the trial is a three week comparison of two topical steroids, I would think that before four years we should have given up.

*Dr. S. Pearse (Parke Davies):*  Anaesthetists often anaesthetise patients who have been on a wide variety of drugs for varying periods of time. When a toxic reaction occurs they really do not know where to start. They do not know which particular drugs are involved, whether the physiology or the pathology are more relevant than the drugs themselves or what was really the cause of the basic reaction. What are your views on this?

*Dr. Harcus:*  This is why I was delighted to be asked to speak about monitoring adverse reactions and not about the assessment of adverse reactions. This is the million dollar question which hangs over nearly all the reports we get. What is the interpretation of the data? In many situations there are so many drugs that the question remains unanswered. The intensive surveillance schemes can help with this problem. They can specifically look at groups of patients who have had a particular drug and see if there is a pattern. The assessment of adverse reactions is an unsatisfactory field because controlled studies of rare events are very difficult.

*Dr. P.G.T. Bye (Schering):*  There is often a good correlation between the incidence and severity of side effects and the blood levels of drug achieved. It is seldom practical to find out what the blood level is in a patient who has an adverse reaction because you do not learn about it in time. If the drug has a long half life you might be able to do something about it if you get an urgent telephone call and the patient is near at hand. Generally it is not possible. You suggested that the drug might be given as a provocative test to assess an adverse reaction. This may not always be feasible. Where feasible the person who gave the drug in the first place might be persuaded to give at least one more dose to the patient. Is it not a good idea to persuade people to do this; and to find out what the half life of the drug is in that particular patient? In this way we might pick up some useful information.

*Dr. Harcus:*  I agree. I think that we should rechallenge where it is ethically acceptable. There is no question of rechallenge with a drug that causes anaphylactic shock. If we do rechallenge, then we should look at every possible factor including blood levels.

*Dr. C. Maxwell (London):*  Mr. Grady, we were very interested in your exhibit from the practolol trial, and were curious to know how the doctor answered when you pointed out that one of the twenty housewives on placebo was male.

*Mr. Grady:*  That is my standard test to find out whether the audience is awake or asleep. Yesterday they were asleep because no one noticed that one of the proformas that I showed had columns 42 and 43 repeated twice due to an error on my part.

*Dr. S. Wynn (CIBA):*  Have you looked at the possibility of using character recognition to read record forms?

*Mr. Grady:*  We looked at marked sensing when it was in its infancy. We found that it did not have anything to offer. We have been using our system for a long time and although we are not complacent, we find it is a satisfactory system. We are fairly heavily committed to it, and have people who are skilled in it with years of expertise. Although we are not averse to looking at other systems, we concentrate on getting on with what we know how to do well.

*Dr. G.A. Poulter (Ortho):*  Mr. Grimshaw, do you invalidate the visual analogue scale if you show the patients what they did previously? Would this get rid of one of your objections to the use of this method?

*Mr. Grimshaw:*  All you succeed in doing is proving to the patient that he is not consistent in his reponse. We have several times gone back to the same intelligent individual, ten minutes after they have filled in the scale, and have said that we have lost the earlier results. They have been asked to repeat the test. We then superimpose the two scales and the result is horrifying. You ought to try it some time. I think it is difficult to justify the use of visual analogue scales in many conditions. Personally I have doubts about the use in the long run of visual analogue scales.

*Dr. R.K. Rondel (Bristol-Meyers):*  What happens if you show them what they scored last week and then ask them to do it again?

*Mr. Grimshaw:* What you are really doing is forcing them into a bracket. You might just as well use semantic differentials and say to them 'your pain was severe last week, how is it this week?'. You are using a scale instead of semantics. Which can the patient understand best? I prefer semantics.

*Dr. R.K. Rondel (Bristol-Meyers):* Mr. Grimshaw, you mentioned the apparent conflict between companies on the publication of results. Journals are not interested in publishing papers that do not show statistically significant results. We have been considering the idea of a journal of negative results. I do not think it will ever happen, but technically we should publish our entire trials programme in some way. It may not be practical but is a solution to your comment.

*Mr. Grimshaw:* I agree with you. One of the greatest disservices to statistics is to enshrine the level of five per cent significance with immortality. There is no such thing at all. The correct way to handle results is to see where the results occur on the frequency distribution, and to work out the probability that they can occur in an extreme portion of the curve. Having determined the probability, you should use your clinical judgement as to whether it is meaningful or not. Statistics is really nothing more than a means of illuminating clinical results. As I have said many times, they do not surpass clinical results in any sense. Hanging on to five per cent significance levels is a real block to progress. There is a great danger in this.

*Dr. S. Wynn (CIBA):* Fisher's exact test results in a substantial loss of power because you are assuming fixed margins. At CIBA we have developed a test which is more powerful and it does not assume fixed margins, which in fact occur rarely in practice. If anyone would like a copy of the programme, they should get in touch with CIBA.

*Mr. Grimshaw:* Thank you. That is a fair comment.

# PART 4
# MODEL SPECIMENS OF CLINICAL TRIALS: CRITERIA

# 16.  Anti-anginal Trials

T. D. V. LAWRIE, W. S. HILLIS, A. TWEDDEL

Coronary heart disease is one of the most common causes of morbidity and mortality in the United Kingdom. This is especially so in young and middle-aged men, where it is the most important single cause of death. Coronary heart disease (CHD) may present as angina pectoris, myocardial infarction, cardiac failure or sudden death. It is therefore not surprising that numerous therapeutic agents have been tried for these clinical manifestations of CHD. This chapter is concerned with reviewing the modern basis for assessing compounds which may be used in the management of angina pectoris. It is primarily concerned with trials aimed at having a therapeutic effect in stable angina pectoris. Unstable angina or pre-infarction angina presents an entirely different problem and is, therefore, outside the scope of this chapter.

Angina pectoris was originally described by Heberden in 1768. He noted its cardinal features, namely location, character, radiation and relation to exercise. The pain is normally substernal, constricting in character, radiating to left arm, less frequently to right arm, is brought on by exercise and is relieved by rest. It is believed to result from an imbalance of myocardial oxygen demand and supply which leads to myocardial ischaemia. Its commonest cause is obstructive atherosclerotic disease of the coronary arteries.

In any anti-anginal trial two important requirements must be met before the trial is designed, the proper selection of cases and the use of adequate techniques for assessment of the compound.

## Selection of cases

In the selection of cases a full clinical history and physical examination is essential. It is important to exclude intra- or extra- cardiac conditions, such as aortic stenosis, thyroid dysfunction or anaemia, because they could invalidate the results of the trial. It is probably essential to separate anginal patients who are normotensive from those who are hypertensive, as this may have important therapeutic implications. Likewise it is desirable to determine whether a prospective candidate for the trial suffers from hyperlipoproteinaemia and whether this is familial or sporadic. Familial hyperlipoproteinaemia tends to be associated with a severe degree of coronary atherosclerosis, even in young individuals, and has a bad prognosis.

The resting electrocardiogram is an important diagnostic investigation in that it may give unequivocal objective evidence of myocardial ischaemia. However, it may be normal in up to 50% of subjects with proven obstructive coronary atherosclerosis and is, therefore, not specific. Exercise electrocardiography is a more sensitive indicator of obstructive coronary atherosclerosis, forms an important part of the investigation of patients entering anti-anginal trials and allows the response to therapy to be assessed. It will be discussed in more detail later.

The definitive investigation which is now essential for patients entering anti-anginal trials is coronary angiography. This diagnostic investigation is now commonplace in all modern cardiological departments.

## Diagram of the Coronary Arteries

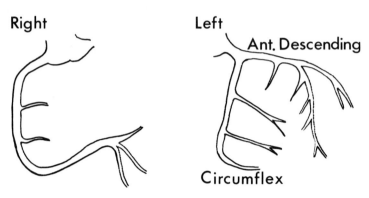

Fig. 16.1 Diagram of the coronary arteries - right and left main coronary arteries. The latter divides into the circumflex and left anterior descending arteries.

The heart is supplied by two main coronary arteries, right and left. The left coronary artery divides soon after its origin into the left anterior descending and circumflex arteries (Fig. 16.1). For practical purposes obstructive coronary atherosclerosis is described as single, double or triple vessel disease depending on the number of major arteries involved (the left main coronary artery, if involved, represents double vessel disease). Involvement of a coronary artery means reduction of the lumen to approximately 60 per cent of its diameter. It is important to note that not all patients giving a typical history of angina pectoris have underlying coronary atherosclerosis. In our own series of 133 cases (Murray *et al.*, 1975) presenting with a typical history of angina pectoris, the angiographic findings were as follows:

| | |
|---|---|
| Normal vessels | 6% |
| Single vessel disease | 25% |
| Double vessel disease | 25% |
| Triple vessel disease | 44% |

Some workers have reported a higher incidence than 6 per cent of patients with normal arteries but with a typical angina history. It is thought that these patients may have coronary artery spasm, small vessel disease, an oxygen dissociation defect or a myocardial metabolic abnormality as the basis for their angina. It is important that these patients be excluded from anti-anginal trials.

The prognosis of patients with angina pectoris varies according to the degree of vessel involvement. The five year mortality (Bruschke, Proudfit and Jones, 1973) is:

| | |
|---|---|
| Single vessel disease | 15% |
| Double vessel disease | 38% |
| Triple vessel disease | 54% |
| Left main coronary artery disease | 57% |

These mortality rates are of importance in trials of angina pectoris, whch are aimed at preventing its complications, and may even modify the results of short-term therapeutic anti-anginal trials.

## Techniques of assessment

Angina pectoris is characterised by symptoms rather than by signs and because of its intrinsic subjective nature has made anti-anginal compounds difficult to evaluate. Therefore, it is important when trying to assess the efficacy of such anti-anginal compounds to use, as far as possible, objective methods of assessment. These should preferably be non-invasive so that they can be repeated several times during the trial without harming the patients.

### Exercise testing

This has become an increasingly popular method of measuring a patient's capacity to work and therefore is suited to measure what anginal patients can do and what effect new compounds may have on exercise tolerance. Tests of dynamic exercise may be classified according to the equipment used, the degree of work load and the end points achieved.

The simple step test is inexpensive as regards equipment, is portable and allows good quality electrocardiographic recordings. The amount of work performed, however, is variable and difficult to standardise. Rhythmical leg work performed by cycling on an upright bicycle ergometer can be readily quantified and associated anxiety and learning difficulties can be minimised by using a 'run in' period. Similar quantitative assessment of work loads can be determined while walking on a motor driven treadmill. At present it is difficult to say which method is preferable. Whether the bicycle ergometer or treadmill is used, 2 to 3 minutes are required at each work load to achieve adequate circulatory adaptation and a plateau in oxygen consumption (Blackmon et al., 1967).

The exercise may be adjusted to achieve submaximal or maximal heart rates. Submaximal exercise is usually used for routine diagnostic stress testing with one or more predetermined end points. These may include a specific duration of work load, oxygen uptake or target heart rate adjusted to 90 per cent of the expected average normal heart rate for age and activity status. Maximal exercise tests are used in anti-anginal trials with individually determined criteria for limiting exercise but it is difficult to determine how closely patients approach their maximum performance.

Chest pain of ischaemic character and distribution must be repeatedly precipitated by the same work load and after the same period of time. As chest pain remains a subjective finding, objective evidence of myocardial ischaemia should be sought in the monitored electrocardiogram, the ST segment depression. Following submaximal exercise the ST segment shift should be greater than 1 mm for a duration of at least 0.08 seconds persisting for 2 to 4 minutes after exercise. These criteria have a sensitivity of 62 per cent for detection and 89 per cent specificity for the exclusion of obstructive coronary atherosclerosis (Martin and McConahay, 1972). The exercise programme used routinely in our exercise laboratory is shown in Table 16.1.

Table 16.1  The basic equipment, the protocol and the end points of exercise testing used in Glasgow Royal Infirmary

| EQUIPMENT | PROTOCOL | END POINTS |
|---|---|---|
| Bicycle ergometer or treadmill | Exercise for 3 minutes at each work load | Target heart rate |
| E.C.G. telemetry system | Work load starts at 300 k.p.m. then increasing | Anginal pain |
| Bipolar chest lead - modified V5 | to 600 k.p.m. and then to 900 k.p.m. (Aim to give three stages of exercise) | Positive E.C.G. |
| Continuous E.C.G. monitoring on oscilloscope | E.C.G. monitoring during and up to 6 minutes after exercising | Dysrhythmias |
| Continuous or intermittent E.C.G. recording | (Facilities available for treating dysrhythmias, syncope or cardiac arrest) | Excessive fatigue or dyspnoea |
| | | Peripheral circulatory insufficiency including claudication |

*Systolic time intervals*

Assessment of cardiac function, in particular left ventricular (LV) function, prefer-ably involves the use of non-invasic techniques. Systolic time intervals, which are ob-tained from simultaneously recorded tracings of the electrocardiogram, phonocardio-gram and carotid pulse tracings can be used for this purpose (Fig. 16.2).

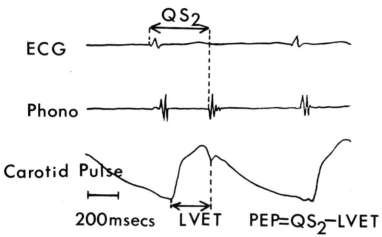

Fig. 16.2 The various systolic time intervals are shown. For a fuller explanation see text.

The intervals measured are:

1. The electromechanical systole or $QS_2$, measured from the Q wave of the electro-cardiogram to the first high frequency deflection of the aortic component of the second heart sound.

2. The left ventricular ejection time (LVET) is measured from the rapid upstroke of the carotid pulse to its incisure.

3. The pre-ejection period (PEP) is measured by subtracting the LVET from the $QS_2$.

4. The PEP/LVET ratio can also be calculated. This ratio has been shown to correlate closely with the LV ejection fraction measured by invasive techniques (Garrard, Weissler and Dodge, 1970).

The PEP is shortened by positive inotropic stimuli such as glycosides, catecholamines or calcium gluconate administration and is prolonged by propranolol (Fig. 16.3) for which a dose response relationship can be demonstrated (Weissler, Harris and Schoenfeld, 1969). The determinants of the PEP are the left ventricular and diastolic pressure (LVEDP) or preload, the rate of rise of the LV pressure and the aortic diastolic press-ure. In conditions where there are minor or no changes in the LVEDP and aortic dia-stolic pressures, then changes in the PEP reflect changes in the contractile state of the left ventricle or LV dp/dt. Therefore, this prolongation or shortening can be used as a physiological 'marker' of pharmacological activity, allowing quantitative and qualitative assessment to be made (Ahmed *et al.*, 1972; Talley, Meyer and McNay, 1971).

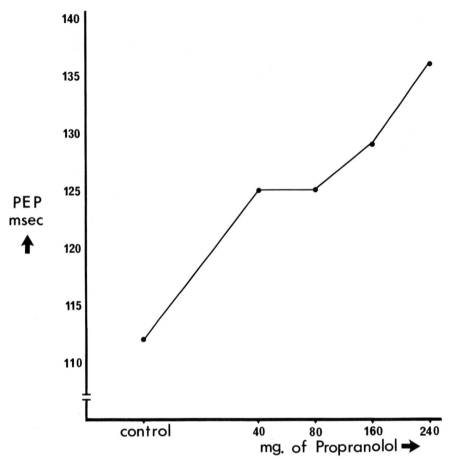

Fig. 16.3 This graph illustrates the lengthening of the PEP with increasing doses of propranolol.

*Echocardiography*

This has been increasingly used in recent years to study the size, shape and contractile state of the left ventricle. Echoes may be recorded simultaneously from the interventricular septum and the posterior wall of the ventricle (Feigenbaum *et al.*, 1969). This allows measurement of the end-diastolic and end-systolic diameters. The end-diastolic and end-systolic volumes may be calculated from established formulae (Troy, Pombo and Rackley, 1972; Popp *et al.*, 1973). Stroke volume, ejection fraction and circumferential fibre shortening may then be derived (Popp and Harrison, 1970; Fortuin *et al.*, 1971; Gibson and Brown, 1973). This method allows serial measurements of these parameters following serial administration of the compound. In some patients with CHD there may be areas of akinesis or dyskinesis of the left ventricle. These abnormalities make volume measurements less accurate using this technique.

*The diary method*

The patient records faithfully each day the frequency of anginal attacks and the consumption of trinitrin tablets. The results of this technique have to be interpreted with caution. An effective anti-anginal compound may not necessarily reduce the frequency of attacks or the number of trinitrin tablets taken because the patient may be able to exercise more rapidly or for a longer time before he develops angina. The method of assessment is, therefore, of limited value unless carried out by reliable witnesses.

*Haemodynamic measurements*

The major determinants of myocardial oxygen consumption include the heart rate, systolic intraventricular pressure and wall tension, the inotropic state of the ventricle and ventricular size. In obstructive coronary atherosclerosis, the 'coronary reserve' is compromised. Coronary blood flow and oxygen delivery cannot be augmented beyond a fixed limit when an increased demand is made on the myocardium. Most therapeutic interventions are aimed at altering favourably the haemodynamic variables upon which myocardial oxygen consumption is dependant (Table 16.2).

Table 16.2 Some of the measurements of left ventricular function obtained at cardiac catheterisation. The compound used in this study was tolamolol.

Haemodynamic & LV function measurements after I.V Tolamolol

|  | control | 5min | 10 min | 15min |
|---|---|---|---|---|
| Heart rate (beats/min) | 81 ± 7 | 62 ± 3 | 66 ± 5 | 69 ± 5 |
| Systolic blood pressure (mmHg) | 123 ± 5 | 117 ± 6 | 118 ± 5 | 113 ± 6 |
| Systemic vascular resistance (dynes$^{-1}$ cm$^{-5}$) | 1547 ± 115 | 1996 ± 171 | 1758 ± 134 | 1578 ± 115 |
| LV end diastolic pressure (mmHg) | 5.3 ± 0.6 | 5.0 ± 1.2 | 5.0 ± 1.1 | 5.0 ± 1.2 |
| LV $dp/dt$ max (mmHg/s) | 1019 ± 57 | 780 ± 53 | 793 ± 49 | 771 ± 56 |

The direct measurement of these variables requires invasive techniques such as cardiac catheterisation. Left ventricular pressures measured by catheter tipped manometers allow changes in the contractile state to be measured and injection of contrast medium allows calculation of the ventricular volumes. The invasive nature of these tests inhibits their use in general anti-anginal trials.

Indirect measurements of myocardial oxygen consumption have been derived using indices which represent some of the major haemodynamic determinants. Such measurements include the double product, heart rate x aortic systolic pressure (Katz and Feinberg, 1958; Jorgensen, Wang and Gobel, 1973);tension time index, the integral of left ventricular pressure during systole x heart rate (Sarnoff, Braunwald and Welch, 1958); the triple product, heart rate x systolic blood pressure x left ventricular ejection time (Epstein *et al.*, 1971). Some of these indices require direct measurement of arterial or left ventricular pressure. Some workers have suggested that the systolic blood pressure might be measured by the cuff technique rather than by invasive techniques. The calculation of the indices of the triple product would allow serial measurements to be carried out and so give indirect, objective evidence of alterations in myocardial oxygen demand and myocardial blood flow following the administrations of anti-anginal compounds. They have provided much information concerning the patho-physiology of angina and its alteration by therapeutic intervention.

### Design of trials

The rational clinical assessment of any new anti-anginal compound requires study in three successive stages. Objective evidence of activity should be gathered at each of these stages:

1. Pharmacodynamic and pharmacokinetic studies must be performed on normal volunteers and patients in the clinical laboratory to confirm animal pharmacology.

2. Wider use on patients can then be undertaken to establish the potential therapeutic usefulness, dosage schedules and possible toxic effects of the compound under investigation.

3. Formal assessment of its therapeutic merits and comparison with other compounds can then be carried out.

The design of the clinical trials will be tailored to the needs of each stage of development, the type of compound being evaluated and the nature and extent of objective measurements performed. Accordingly, two types of human studies have been developed:

a. *Pharmacological experiments* in which the individual is subjected to special investigations, often using complex measuring techniques such as have been described under haemodynamic investigations.

b. *Therapeutic experiments* in which the measurements made on individuals are of a simpler nature, e.g. exercise testing. Groups of patients can then be treated in different ways to provide data for comparison of different compounds.

First it is desirable to assess an anti-anginal compound in an acute study, prescribing the compound in intravenous, oral or sublingual form. The exercise test is the usual procedure adopted for objective assessment of the efficacy of the drug - the protocol for such exercise testing is given above (Table 16.1). It is important to standardise the procedure by having a 'run-in' period to allow the patients to become thoroughly familiar with the exercise procedure; and also to make certain that any improvement in exercise tolerance is due to the effect of the compound rather than training. The minimum for the 'run-in' period is four weekly visits. It must be appreciated that the end point is chest pain, which is subjective. This makes it all the more important that the patients selected for the trial are suffering from stable angina and that the amount of exercise required to produce chest pain is reproducible over a period of days, weeks or a few months. Repetitive exercise testing in any one individual should be standardised, i.e. carried out at the same time of the day, in the same environment and under the same work load.

The duration of the trial is of considerable importance. If it is too long then the effect of climate (summer v. winter) may significantly alter results. Furthermore, the natural progress of the underlying disease (again depending on whether single, double or triple vessel disease is present) may affect the outcome of the trial. It is possible to offset these factors by restricting the period of treatment to a few weeks on any one drug or placebo in random order. Such cycles can be repeated if necessary. At the other end of the scale the period of assessment of the compound can be too short. Three months is probably the minimum period for a short term trial.

The dosage of the compound may influence the results of a therapeutic trial, according to whether a fixed or a variable dose is used. This has been demonstrated very well in the studies of β-adrenoreceptor blocking compounds in angina pectoris. Different individuals require different doses of a β-blocking compound to produce the same degree of beta-blockade, as measured by the degree of bradycardia produced. The dosage of a compound may be influenced by the height, weight and body build of the patient. For this reason a variable rather than a fixed dose may be preferable in any anti-anginal trial. Fixed or variable dose trials in which all the patients receive the same dosage or have their dose individually adjusted, can be carried out but these tend to be complex and difficult to handle. Blood levels are not necessarily helpful in this context as has been shown with propranolol.

In summarising the present position of anti-anginal trials there is little doubt that considerable advances have been made in recent years. With the introduction of coronary angiography the selection of cases has improved significantly. Pharmacodynamic and pharmacokinetic studies have led to a better understanding of the absorption and metabolism of compounds and dosage schedules have been put on a more rational basis. Techniques for measuring the efficacy of anti-anginal compounds have also improved. Although the non-invasive techniques of exercise testing, systolic time intervals and echocardiography lack the precision of the more sophisticated, invasive haemodynamic techniques, they still give useful information about the actions of compounds under investigation. Further developments of non-invasive techniques can be expected, thus improving the overall quality of anti-anginal trials.

# REFERENCES

Ahmed, S.S. Levinson, G.E., Schwarz, C.J. & Ettinger, P.O. (1972) Systolic time intervals as measures of the contractile state of the left ventricular myocardium in man. *Circulation*, **46**, 559 - 572.

Blackmon, J.R., Rowell, L.B., Kennedy, J.W.,Twiss, R.D. & Conn, R.D. (1967) Physiological significance of maximal oxygen intake in pure mitral stenosis. *Circulation*, **36**, 497 - 510.

Bruschke, A.V.G. Proudfit, W.L. & Jones, F.M. (1973) Progress study of 590 consecutive non-surgical cases of coronary disease followed 5 - 9 years. *Circulation*, **47**, 1147 - 1154.

Epstein, S.E., Redwood, D.R., Goldstein, R.E.,Beiser, D., Rosing, D.R., Glancy, D.L., Reis, R.L. & Stinson, E.B. (1971). Angina pectoris: pathophysiology, evaluation and treatment. *Annals of Internal Medicine*, **75**, 263 - 296.

Feigenbaum, H., Wolfe, S.B., Popp, R.L., Haine, C.L. & Dodge, H.T. (1969) Correlation of ultrasound with angiocardiography in measuring left ventricular volume. *American Journal of Cardiology,* **23,** 111.

Fortuin, N.J., Hooo, W.P., Sherman, M.E., & Craige, E. (1971) Determination of left ventricular volumes with ultrasound. *Circulation,* **44,** 575 - 584.

Garrard, C.L., Weissler, A.M. & Dodge, H.T. (1970) The relationship of alterations in systolic time intervals to ejection fraction in patients with cardiac disease. *Circulation,* **42,** 455 - 462.

Gibson, D & Brown, D. (1973) Measurement of instantaneous left ventricular dimension and filling rate with echocardiography. *British Heart Journal,* **35,** 1141 - 1149.

Jorgensen, C.R., Wang, K. & Gobel, F.L. (1973) Effect of propranolol on myocardial oxygen consumption and its haemodynamic correlates during upright exercise. *Circulation,* **48,** 1173 - 1182.

Katz, L.N. & Feinberg, H. (1958) The relation of cardiac effort to myocardial oxygen consumption and coronary flow. *Circulation Research,* **6,** 656.

Martin, C.M. & McConahay, D.R. (1972) Maximal treadmill exercise electrocardiography correlation with coronary arteriography and cardiac haemodynamics. *Circulation,* **44,** 956 - 963.

Murray, R.G., Tweddel, A., Third, J.L.H.C., Hutton, I., Hillis, W.S., Lorimer, A.R. & Lawrie, T.D.V. (1975) Relation between extent of coronary artery disease and severity of hyperlipoproteinaemia. *British Heart Journal,* **37** (12), 1205 - 1210.

Popp, R.L. & Harrison, D.C. (1970) Ultrasonic cardiac echography for determining stroke volume and valvular regurgitation. *Circulation,* **42,** 493 - 502.

Popp, R.L., Alderman, E.L., Brown, O.R. & Harrison, D.C. (1973) Sources of error in calculation of left ventricular volume. *American Journal of Cardiology,* **31,** 152.

Sarnoff, S.J., Braunwald, E. & Welch, G.R. (1958) Haemodynamic determinants of oxygen consumption of the heart with special reference to the tension time index. *American Journal of Physiology,* **192,** 148 - 157.

Talley, R.C., Meyer, J.F. & McNay, J.L. (1971) Evaluation of pre-ejection period as an estimate of myocardial contractility in dogs. *American Journal of Cardiology,* **27,** 384.

Troy, B.L., Pombo, J. & Rackley, C.E. (1972) Measurement of left ventricular wall thickness and mass by electrocardiography. *Circulation,* **45,** 602 - 611.

Weissler, A.M., Harris, W.S. & Schoenfeld, C.D. (1969) Bedside techniques for the evaluation of ventricular function in man. *American Journal of Cardiology,* **23,** 577 - 583.

# 17. Clinical Trials of Antibiotics

D. S. REEVES

This chapter is an account of antibiotic clinical trials based on my own experience. Only trials of treatment of bacterial infection will be discussed, excluding antituberculous therapy, I shall concentrate on the factors unique to antibiotic trials.

## Objectives of the clinical trial

The early clinical study of a new antibacterial drug should be done in hospital under close supervision. It is then possible to satisfy the four principal objectives: To determine efficacy in terms of cure or prevention of infection; to assess pharmacology, tolerance and toxicity. Investigate the drug by itself first. Comparative trials come later using agents suggested by study of the initial results.

Trials in hospital also permit study of the reaction to the antibiotic of patients who have the more severe pathology. Tolerance may be less in particular patients, with mild disease or in the elderly. For example we found that a penicillin ester was poorly tolerated in pregnancy. This discovery in the clinical trial stage allowed valuable advice on dosing to be given.

## Clinical material and entry to trial

It is rare to attempt treatment of a single bacterial species except where it is the sole pathogen by definition, such as gonococcal urethritis or typhoid fever. Usually patients present with a complex of signs and symptoms indicating an infection which could be caused by a variety of bacterial species; examples are urinary infection, chest infection, or meningitis. Bacteriological definition of the cause is essential. Comparison with other trials of the drug can be made if the clinical material is homogeneous and defined.

Some typical infections are given in Table 17.1, with the comparative importance of various investigations to determine entry to the trial. Usually bacteriological proof is required. Inclusion is impossible without it if symptoms are not specific (for example, bacteraemia) or absent (asymptomatic bacteriuria), or because the diagnosis involves a specific pathogen (gonorrhoea). Bacteriological confirmation is not always possible, for example in exacerbations of chronic bronchitis. A recognised bacterial pathogen is isolated from only 40 to 60 per cent of patients (May, 1972). There are also difficulties in interpreting the true significance of these isolates.

## Criteria of infection

Criteria of infection must be satisfied before a patient is put into a trial. The main

163

Table 17.1 Criteria of entry for some typical infections treated in clinical trials of antibiotics

| 'Syndrome' | Microbiological investigation by culture | other | Clinical assessment | Other tests |
|---|---|---|---|---|
| Acute symptomatic urinary infection | + | urinary cells | + | — |
| Asymptomatic bacteriuria | | | | |
| (i) pregnancy | + | — | — | — |
| (ii) non-pregnancy | + | — | — | radiology localisation of infection |
| Gonococcal urethritis | + | — | + | — |
| Surgical wound infection | + | — | ++ | — |
| Upper respiratory infection | | | | |
| (i) sore throat | + | ⎰ ASO titre / 'virus' titres | + | — |
| (ii) middle ear/sinus | +/– | ⎱ virus culture | ++ | — |
| Lower respiratory infection | +/– | 'virus' titres | ++ | radiology lung function tests sputum purulence and volume |
| Bacteraemia | + | — | + | — |
| Acute osteomyelitis | +/– | — | ++ | radiology |
| Enteric fever | + | serology | + | — |

+ culture essential; clinical assessment useful for determination of efficacy
+/– cultural diagnosis not always possible
++ clinical assessment essential before entry

criterion of infection is the isolation of a pathogenic organism from the appropriate specimen. With normally sterile material, such as cerebrospinal fluid or blood, quantitation of the isolate is not necessary; provided it is a bacterium associated with the disease. From other material, repeated isolation may be necessary and some form of quantitation used. The classic example is asymptomatic bacteriuria. This is usually taken as being present when there are two successive cultures of the same bacterial species in the urine at more than 100,000 organism/ml ($10^8/1$) (Kass, 1962).

Bacterial isolation is slow. Symptomatic patients may need treatment before the results of cultures are available. If nothing is isolated, it may then be necessary to exclude the patient from the study of efficacy. These patients should not be completely excluded because information can be obtained on pharmacology, tolerance and toxicity. For example, with acute urinary infection, the clinician takes a urine specimen and prescribes an antimicrobial. About half these patients have significant bacteriuria: But it is not practical and probably not necessary to call a patient back after 2 to 3 days therapy and tell them to stop the treatment. The more cynical of us reckon that the patient would have stopped anyway when the symptoms subsided.

Clinical examination is sometimes essential. For example, the isolation of *Staphlococcus aureus* does not necessarily indicate w wound infection. Clinical criteria such as erythema, exudation and induration must be fulfilled. In acute osteomyelitis an organism may never be isolated from the bone lesion, or may be isolated from blood culture alone. Diagnosis will have to be made on clinical and radiological grounds alone in about one third of patients (Blockey and McAllister, 1972).

Symptoms and signs of infection can also form part of the assessment of efficacy. This may be in the grossest terms like survival, or crude as with elevation of fever in typhoid (Sardeasai, Karandikar and Harshe, 1973). Many symptoms resolve spontaneously, as in acute urinary infection (Brooks, Garrett and Hollihead, 1972). The effect of the drug may not be clear unless a placebo control is used. This may not be ethical, as in gonorrhoea!

A record of the clinical history is essential for age, weight, primary diagnosis and any other pathology which might influence the outcome of therapy. For example, a bladder tumour or neurogenic bladder might affect treatment of a urinary tract infection. Special tests may be necessary to improve the homogeneity of groups of patients. Notable examples are those to localise urinary infection to the upper or lower urinary tract (Reeves and Brumfitt, 1968).

## Criteria of cure

When the criterion of infection is bacteriological, the criterion of cure is the eradication of the original organism. If the specific pathogen is not a commensal, there are no problems. Reinfection does not necessarily indicate a failure of treatment. Reinfection may be with the same bacterial species, but a different organism only distinguishable by intraspecies typing, for example O-serotyping or phage typing (Fig. 17.1). Special facilities are required (Brumfitt and Reeves, 1969). A centre without such facilities can still undertake a well designed study as typing is only necessary in a few patients. Failure of eradication is shown by persistence of the original organism during therapy, even in low numbers, and relapse within a week following therapy. Reinfection may occur at any time. An infection present four

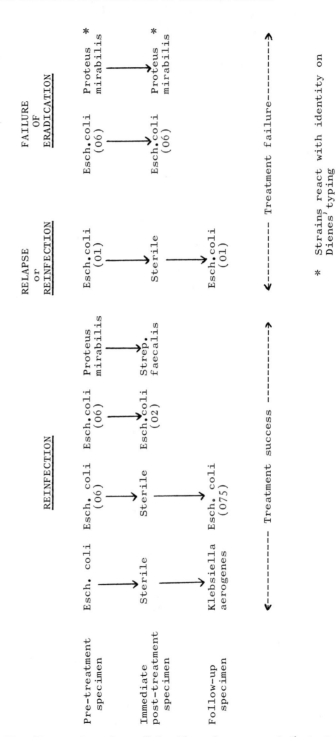

Fig. 17.1  Use of intraspecies typing to distinguish varying responses to the treatment of urinary infections.

weeks after stopping treatment but not present a few days after treatment is almost certainly a reinfection (Grüneberg, Leigh and Brumfitt, 1969).

The timing of follow up specimens depends on the known interval before relapse due to failure of therapy becomes apparent. Drug in blood, cerebrospinal fluid, sputum, urine and other specimens taken during therapy may cause inhibition of growth. Laboratory techniques should allow for this. Bacterial isolation after therapy may be more difficult than before therapy because of the smaller number of organisms in the lesion. Multiple specimens may be desirable to ensure that eradication has occurred.

When no cultural diagnosis was made before treatment, cure must be assessed by other means. In chest infections this will mainly be by clinical criteria, sputum volume and purulence, and radiology. Lung function tests are, in our experience, not particularly helpful. Base line tests before therapy are not usually possible in the more ill patients (Reeves and Thomas, in press). In asymptomatic bacteriuria clinical criteria are valueless.

## Quantitative determination of microbial susceptibility

Organisms should be kept to determine sensitivity to the test drug. The decision to include a patient will usually rely on the result of a sensitivity disc test. These tests are subject to error and some organisms may be resistant when reexamined. This would be important in the assessment of efficacy.

When two drugs are being used in combination (for example, cotrimoxazole) the in vitro examination of the sensitivity of the infecting organism is more complex. It should include minimal inhibitory concentrations of the individual agents and also combined tests for synergy (Grüneberg and Kolbe, 1969).

## Pharmacological assessment

All new antibiotics should also be assessed pharmacologically in patients. Studies in human volunteers are no substitute for investigation under working conditions. The pharmacology may be different because of primary disease. Patients are a heterogenous group, therefore a wide scatter of results is to be expected. In particular, oral absorption is very variable, partially due to the difficulty of controlling dosing in relation to meals. Unless one stands over the patient, it is not certain that the drug is even taken, let along at any particular time. Pharmacological studies are exacting because of the need to take blood samples at particular times. This is not easy for laboratory staff and almost impossible for most clinicians. It is often necessary to take samples over a weekend. Timed urine collections may be incomplete; a knowledge of the particular nursing staff is invaluable for assessing this factor.

Even when the samples are safely collected there are further problems. Some antibiotics are not stable and although assay of batches of samples is desirable for convenience and accuracy, deterioration can occur with storage. We now assay all samples as soon as possible.

Tactfully enquire about the accuracy of assays done in the investigator's laboratory. This is particularly necessary when quantitative information on bioavailability is needed. If the question 'what is your per cent accuracy at 95 per cent confidence limits?' produces a bemused expression then beware. It is unlikely that the investigator has even considered that his assays may be inaccurate. Microbiological assay performed by most laboratories is less than $\pm$ 25 per cent accurate at 95 per cent confidence limits. It is thus not acceptable for controlling aminoglycoside therapy let alone pharmacological measurements (Reeves and Bywater, 1975).

### Toxicological assessment

The battery of standard laboratory screening tests required before, during and after therapy should present no problem to most hospital laboratories. Trials of some antibiotics require special tests. With aminoglycosides clinical tests of auditory and vestibular function can be of use although they will miss the high tone deafness and other minor toxic responses. Audiometry and objective tests of vestibular integrity such as electronystagmography are essential for scientific assessment.

While not 'toxicity' in the usual sense, changes induced in body flora by antibiotics may need to be monitored. In long term prophylactic therapy for urinary infection, reinfection may occur with organisms from the bowel selected by their resistance to treatment. Some drugs have more potential than others for causing such selection. Pre- and post-treatment faecal cultures may reveal this (Lincoln, Lidin-Janson and Winberg, 1972).

Special groups of patients may require additional monitoring for possible toxic effects. If it is necessary to give a new antimicrobial drug during pregnancy, the baby must be examined for possible damage. Antimicrobial drugs given late in pregnancy might cause problems in neonatal life by displacing bilirubin bound to serum protein (Sutherland and Light, 1965). Because of the immaturity of detoxifying mechanisms and renal function, antibiotic elimination requires special attention in neonates (Yaffe and Rane, 1971). Additional toxicological and pharmacological tests may be required.

Drug interactions may occur by stimulation of microsomal liver enzymes as with rifampicin and the contraceptive pill. There may be interference with metabolism causing enhanced activity of the second drug (Christensen, Hansen and Kristensen, 1963). The administration of a second drug may substantially shorten the plasma half life of an antibiotic, as with barbiturates and doxycycline (Neuvonen and Penttila, 1974). General tests for enzyme induction such as decrease of antipyrine half life or increase of D-glucaric acid excretion may be indicated (Hunter, 1974).

### Assessment of tolerance

The occurrence of reactions attributable to therapy must be recorded. The investigator should visit the patient personally at least twice during a short course of therapy. Reporting by third parties cannot be relied upon. I have known both the patient and his nurses miss the presence of a rash. Continuity of assessment from the pretherapy visit onwards is useful to avoid over or under recording.

To a laboratory based trialist working with other doctors' patients, good drug tolerance is a desirable feature. Patients who complain vociferously of pills which cause vomiting or of injections causing pain are bound to sour one's relationhip with the clinician; and the nursing staff become uncooperative.

### Comparative trials

These follow a successful initial assessment. They may pose many difficulties in trial design. When treatment is commenced without sensitivity testing, the drug for comparison must have a similar spectrum of activity so as to satisfy ethical criteria. It would therefore take a large number of patients to demonstrate any significant difference between the two drugs, even when the patients form a reasonably homogeneous group. In asymptomatic infections sensitivity testing can be carried out before the patient is put into the trial. But this poses problems because the level set *in vitro* for 'sensitivity' may vary between drugs and may still be under investigation for the new drug. Resistant organisms occur in complicated urinary infections making comparison between drugs of differing spectra nearly impossible. When a series of clinical trials with new antibiotics were carried out in hospital patients after sensitivity testing, the cure rates were similar, despite varying doses and routes of administration (Table 17.2).

It is not always ethical to compare two widely differing drugs or a new drug with placebo. For example, neither kanamycin nor carbenicillin could be compared with gentamicin as initial treatment for presumptive bacteraemia since each drug has a different spectrum. There are exceptions such as the comparison of amoxycillin and chloramphenicol in typhoid fever (Pillay, Adams and North-Coombes, 1975) or clindamycin and fusidic acid in acute osteomyelitis. In each case the sensitivity of the infecting organism to both drugs is known.

Double blind trials may be difficult to design practically and are not always necessary. The criteria of infection and cure based on laboratory investigation are unreasonably objective. The investigator should be blind when the relative tolerance of drugs is being studied. The assessor should be independent from the main investigator.

## Adequate staffing

Clinical trials of antibiotics should be undertaken by the clinician looking after the patients but this may be unsatisfactory. As clinicians have many demands on their time, it is not surprising that most antibiotic trials are conducted by a microbiologist. Those doctors who have never done a clinical trial rarely appreciate how much work is needed to obtain complete data. The admission of a patient to an antibiotic trial is time consuming. The doctor must discuss the proposed trial with the patient, examine him and complete the record sheet. He should discuss the details with the clinician in whose care the patient is. He will probably have to take all the blood specimens at the right time himself. The ward sister will have to be persuaded to collect urine samples. The patient with serious infection should be visited at least daily so that progress can be assessed. Lack of progress may warrant abandoning the trial drug.

It is essential to dedicate a medical member of the laboratory staff to a trial when patients are not the clinical responsibility of the investigator. He should be available twenty four hours a day to accept patients offered for the trial. If side effects occur the investigator must be available to discuss them with the clinician otherwise the treatment will probably be stopped.

## Trials outside hospital

Not all clinical trials of antibiotics require elaborate monitoring of pharmacology and toxicity. Well tested drugs can be investigated for efficacy and tolerance in general practice. If the trial is to be objective, it is important to make proper arrangements for bacterial cultures.

Table 17.2   Cure rates of urinary infections in hospital patients in a series of antibiotic trials, Southmead Hospital, 1973 - 76

| Antibiotic | Dose | Days | Route of administration | Cured/treated (%) | Reference |
|---|---|---|---|---|---|
| Ticarcillin | 1 gram 6 hourly | 7 | IM | 13/16 (81%) | 1 |
| Cephacetrile | 1 gram 12 hourly | 5 | IM | 16/21 (76%) | 2 |
| Carfecillin | 1 gram 8 hourly | 7 | oral | 21/35 (60%) | 3 |
| Pivmecillinam | 400 mg 6 hourly | 7 | oral | 29/35 (83%) | 4 |
| Talampicillin | 750 mg 12 hourly | 7 | oral | 29/38 (76%) | 5 |

1. Wise and Reeves, 1974

2. Wise, Reeves and Hepburn, 1974

3. Wilkinson et al., 1975

4. Wise et al., 1976

5. Leigh et al. (in press).

Some diseases occur predominantly in outpatients. Asymptomatic bacteriuria in pregnancy requires treatment. It has been the testing ground for many antibiotics particularly because spontaneous resolution of infection is rare (Williams *et al.*, 1968), unlike acute symptomatic urinary infection. Almost every antibiotic on the market showing appropriate *in vitro* activity has been tested in gonorrhoea. This demonstrates the enthusiasm of veneriologists and the lack of satisfactory treatment. The main difficulties are following up patients and distinguishing reinfection from failure of eradication, because there is no strain typing method for the gonococcus. Cultural diagnosis is essential, particularly in female patients.

### Support from the industry

There are two main types of support for investigators from the pharmaceutical industry: Advice, and providing resources. Antibiotic trials are usually of simple design but the investigator may not appreciate just how much effort the protocol requires. If trials are going to start and keep going, it is important that the investigator knows the difficulties without being put off. The protocol should be as simple as is compatible with obtaining the information required. The investigator's morale may be broken by trying to obtain difficult data.

For antibiotic trials undoubtedly the most precious resource is medical time. Although expensive, money to support a junior medical post may be the best way to ensure a rapid and effective trial. There are often junior medical staff between jobs who are keen to do a trial which will provide them with a publication. Extra use of technical, laboratory and secretarial time is not great since much would have been done as part of routine care. Occasionally payment for a few hours of evening or weekend work is required.

### Conclusion

The value of antibiotics in the treatment of infections is determined by clinical trials. Initial trials are best done in hospital so that the strict criteria of infection and cure can be satisfied by bacteriological control. The condition of hospital patients is different from that of volunteers. Early information on pharmacological behaviour in disease and on drug interaction can be obtained. Close supervision is important for the detection of adverse reactions. The required monitoring is extravagant on medical time. This may be a critical factor in the satisfactory commission of a model protocol. Some infections are found almost entirely in outpatients but even in general practice adequate bacteriological monitoring is essential.

REFERENCES

Blockey, N.J. & McAllister, T.A. (1972) Antibiotics in acute osteomyelitis in children. *Journal of Bone and Joint Surgery*, **54b**, 299 - 309.

Brooks, D., Garrett, G.. & Hollihead, R. (1972) Sulphadimidine, co-trimoxazole, and a placebo in the management of symptomatic urinary tract infection in general practice. *Journal of the Royal College of General Practitioners,* **22,** 695 - 703.

Brumfitt, W. & Reeves, D.S. (1969) Recent developments in the treatment of urinary tract infection. *Journal of Infectious Diseases,* **120,** 61 - 81.

Christensen, L.K., Hansen, J.M. & Kristensen, M. (1963) Sulphaphenazole-induced hypoglycaemic attacks in tolbutamide-treated diabetes. *Lancet,* **ii,** 1298 - 1301.

Grüneberg, R.N. & Kolbe, R. (1969) Trimethoprim in the treatment of urinary infection in hospital. *British Medical Journal,* **1,** 545 - 547.

Grüneberg, R.N. Leigh, D.A. & Brumfitt, W. (1969) *Escherichia coli* serotypes in urinary tract infections: studies in domicillary, antenatal and hospital practice. In *Urinary Tract Infection,* ed. O'Grady, F & Brumfitt, W. Pages 68 - 79. London: Oxford.

Hunter, J. (1974) Enxyme induction and medical treatment. *Journal of the Royal College of Physicians,* **8,** 163 - 174.

Kass, E.H. (1962) Pyelonephritis and bacteriuria. A major problem in preventative medicine. *Annals of Internal Medicine,* **56,** 46.

Leigh, D.A., Reeves, D.S., Simmons, K., Thomas, A.L. & Wilkinson, P.J. (1976) Studies with talampicillin, a new derivative of ampicillin. *British Medical Journal* (in press).

Lincoln, K., Lidin-Janson, G. & Winberg, J. (1972) Faecal and periurethral flora after oral administration of sulphonamide, nitrofurantoin and nalidixic acid. *Acta Paediatrica Scandinavica,* **61,** 643 - 647.

May, J.R. (1972) *The Chemotherapy of Chronic Bronchitis and Allied Disorders.* London: English Universities Press. Page 11.

Neuvonen, P.J. & Penttila, O. (1974) Interaction between doxycycline and barbiturates. *British Medical Journal,* **1,** 535 - 536.

Pillay, N., Adams, E.B. & North-Coombes, D. (1975) Comparative trial of amoxycillin and chloramphenicol in treatment of typhoid fever in adults. *Lancet,* **ii,** 333 - 334.

Reeves, D.S. & Brumfitt, W. (1968) Localisation of urinary tract infection. In *Urinary Tract Infection,* ed. O'Grady, F. & Brumfitt, W. Pages 53 - 67; London: Oxford.

Reeves, D.S. & Bywater, M.J. (1975) Quality control of serum gentamicin assays - experience of national surveys. *Journal of Antimicrobial Chemotherapy,* **1,** 103 - 116.

Reeves, D.S. & Thomas, A.L. (1976) Lower respiratory infections treated with cephacetrile. *Infection.* (in press).

Sardeasai, H.V., Karandikar, R.S. & Harshe, R.G. (1973) Comparative trial of co-trimoxazole and chloramphenicol in typhoid fever. *British Medical Journal,* **1,** 82 - 83.

Sutherland, J.M. & Light I.J. (1965) The effects of drugs upon the developing foetus. *Paediatric Clinics of North America.* **12,** 781 - 806.

Wilkinson, P.J., Reeves, D.S., Wise, R. & Allen, J.T. (1975) Volunteer and clinical studies with carfecillin: a new orally administered ester of carbenicillin. *British Medical Journal,* **ii,** 250 - 252.

Williams, J.D., Reeves, D.S., Condie, A.P., Franklin, I.S.N., Leigh, D.A. & Brumfitt, W. (1968) The treatment of bacteriuria in pregnancy. In *Urinary Tract Infection.* ed. O'Grady, F. & Brumfitt, W. Pages 160 - 168. London: Oxford.

Wise, R & Reeves, D.S. (1974) Clinical and laboratory investigations on ticarcillin, an anti-pseudomonal antibiotic. *Chemotherapy,* **20,** 45 - 51.

Wise, R., Reeves, D.S. & Hepburn, P.R. (1974) Cephacetrile, a new cephalosporin, in the treatment of urinary tract infections. *Chemotherapy,* **20,** 177 - 182.

Wise, R., Reeves, D.S., Symonds, J.M. & Wilkinson, P.J. (1976) A clinical investigation of pivmecillinam. A novel $\beta$-lactam antibiotic in the treatment of urinary tract infections. *Chemotherapy,* **22,** 335 - 339.

Yaffe, S.F. & Rane, A. (1971) Developmental aspects of pharmacokinetics. *Acta Pharmacologica et Toxicologica.* **29,** Suppl. 3, 240 - 249.

# 18.   The Designing of Oral Contraceptive Trials

P. G. T. BYE

The evaluation of oral contraceptives demonstrates more clearly than any other kind of drug trial the gulf that lies between what is desirable and what is attainable.

The investigator of oral contraceptives greatly envies the laboratory worker with his thousands of caged subjects copulating to order. In humans we have not even been able to establish the right test conditions for answering such questions as: for how many days should additional precautions, if any, be taken when starting the pill; what sort of errors of tablet taking are compatible with retention of contraceptive effect; is it really necessary to use additional precautions when changing from one oral contraceptive to another containing smaller amounts of hormones? Every day, pronouncements on these matters are made by family planning doctors, yet not one of them is based on firm scientific evidence. To understand the design of oral contraceptive trials one must first appreciate their limitations.

### Efficacy

The first questions usually asked about a new oral contraceptive concern its efficacy. In most drug trials, we can assume that if the majority of tablets have been taken the effect of the drug can be interpreted. Errors of tablet taking will occur, but unused tablets can be collected and allowance made for the lower dosage taken. But protection from pregnancy requires more or less continued use of oral contraceptives. A patient may take her tablets flawlessly for all but a crucial day or two in a study lasting a year. If she should become pregnant the effect on the efficacy data will be out of all proportion to the magnitude of the error. Conception is a fairly rare event in any contraceptive trial, and a single pregnancy can have a striking effect on the total figures. Therefore, in order to assess what degree of protection a pill is capable of giving we should aim to obtain correct information about tablet taking by getting the patient to keep an accurate daily record. Patients have often been seen filling in weeks at a time of such records while waiting to see the trialist.

If a woman becomes pregnant and admits that she has omitted tablets we can believe her, since she is unlikely to have any motive for lying about it, but the converse is not true. When pregnancy has occurred as a result of a foolish error on her part she has an obvious motive for concealing it. By contrast, such gross omissions of consecutive tablets are sometimes admitted that it is hard to believe that they were true errors. The desire of many women to have more babies, which they may be unwilling to admit to their husbands, their doctors or even themselves may be almost the total determinant of the pregnancy rate.

Trials have been done in the USA (not with oral contraceptives) in which the daily dose of drug had to be removed from a special container. The consequent movement of a small radioactive source over a strip of film inside the container showed any variation in the intervals between extractions of drug from the machine. These gadgets are too expensive to use in trials of the size usual with oral contraceptives, and do not ensure that the drug has been taken. However, assuming that we have accurate information about omitted tablets, how much use is it to us? Since the bleeding during oral contraception is artificially induced, and the duration of pregnancy is variable, we cannot accurately date any conceptions that occur. Since pregnancy may happen without errors of tablet taking, it is possible that pregnancy may result from ovulation occurring close to an admitted error but not actually caused by it. Therefore, even if we could be sure that coitus happened at the same time as an error of tablet-taking, it would still not be possible to ascribe a pregnancy with certainty to that error. Moreover, information given by patients about coitus is probably highly inaccurate, and if a record of coitus is requested many women (and even doctors) refuse to participate in the trial. Therefore, no attempt is made to record coitus in many investigations.

Some idea of method effectiveness is obtained by excluding all pregnancies starting during incorrectly taken courses of tablets (as indicated by a lack of subsequent bleeding and by a positive pregnancy test). But this does not discriminate accurately between method failures and patient failures. It may be thought pointless to try, since errors of tablet taking will occur with any self administered drug, and that we need be concerned only with use effectiveness. This is a valid argument if we are not comparing pills but merely want to determine that the failure rate is of an acceptable order. However, comparisons of efficacy between different pills will always be attempted. Such comparisons should be made on the same population, when factors other than the pharmacological properties of the pill play such a large part in determining not only use effectiveness, but also method effectiveness.

Assuming we obtain an estimate of the pregnancy rate, divided into patient failures and method failures, can we conclude from this that product A is more effective than product B? The chance is remote. When a statistician is asked about the appropriate sample size for assessing efficacy in an oral contraceptive trial, what he tells us is daunting. If two pregnancies occur in 5000 trial cycles, this is a pregnancy rate of about 0.5 per hundred woman-years. Statistically, there is a 95 per cent chance that the true pregnancy rate in the population from which the sample was drawn would be between 0.01 and 1.7 per hundred woman-years. Such is the effect of one rare event, that even with very large numbers of cycles, the limits are still wide. Even if there are no pregnancies in a trial of 5000 cycles, the 'true' pregnancy rate may be almost as high as one per hundred woman-years. This degree of uncertainty would still exist if we were able to verify by direct observation that every tablet entered every subject's stomach at the correct time. Hines and Goldzieher (1969) calculated that to show a difference in method failure rate between two pills that was significant at the 5 per cent level, hundreds of thousands ot even millions of cycles would be required. Therefore, trials of oral contraceptives must start with the recognition that the most important property of the pill is doomed to fall short of that sine qua non of the modern clinical trials, the test of statistical significance.

Actually, we do not expect to improve on the present level of efficacy with any method that depends on daily self administration. Since oral contraceptives are so much more reliable than any other method, a minor inferiority of efficacy as compared with previous pills would still leave a new pill more effective than any other method. We assume that if a new pill is markedly less reliable than older ones some suspision of it may become apparent in a clinical trial of reasonable size, even if the difference is not statistically significant. Instead, we are more interested in other aspects of the pill's performance.

### Other aspects

What are the other aspects? One is the pattern of bleeding. To assess cycle control, we want information about each subject's bleeding pattern before the trial. In practical terms it is usually possible to record only the cycle before starting to take the new pill; but Chiazze et al. (1968) found that two out of three healthy women had cycles that varied as much as six days in length, so a single cycle may not be representative. The patient can be asked about the extremes of variability over a designated period, which should be long enough to include variations but not too long for recollection. Unfortunately, recollection is highly unreliable. I found that about sixty per cent of the pretrial cycles proved to be outside the limits previously stated by the patients. Women commonly believe that their cycles are as regular as clockwork. Only those few who keep their own records know this to be untrue. It may be sufficient merely to ask them whether or not their cycle previously has been regular or irregular (without attempting to define the terms). The common belief may lead to their describing the cycles as irregular only when the irregularity is gross, which is probably all that we need to know. This approach has proved useful in my own company. Separate cycle analysis has shown a markedly greater degree of cycle irregularity while taking an oral contraceptive in the group who described their pretrial cycles as irregular.

There are big cultural differences in attitudes to the bleeding pattern. One might expect women to welcome a reduction in menstrual loss, but there is a widespread belief that menstruation purges the body of impurities. This belief may inhibit acceptance of a method that reduces blood loss. Conversely, prolonged bleeding restricts opportunities for coitus. It also extends the period during which Moslem women are ritually unclean and may not prepare food. The importance of bleeding varies from culture to culture. One can draw conclusions about its acceptability only in respect of the cultural group in which the trial is carried out. The difference in women's opinions about the bleeding pattern make it particularly important that we should have accurate information about it. Women must be asked to keep a daily record.

The only easily comprehensible classification of menstruation is into 'bleeding' (requiring sanitary protection) and 'spotting' (requiring no sanitary protection). This distinction is likely to be made by all subjects at a fairly consistent level in a given cultural group. Nowadays no investigator seems to attempt further subdivision of the record of daily bleeding. Any more sophisticated subdivision of bleeding will not have absolute comparability.

Hallberg et al. (1966) asked a group of women to describe their menstrual loss as heavy, moderate or light, and at the same time to collect their sanitary towels in plastic bags. The blood loss was calculated by extracting the iron content of the bags.

There was no correlation whatsoever between the women's menstrual loss and the way they described it. Hallberg's method cannot be applied to a large scale clinical trial. We attempted an objective assessment by asking patients to record the number of sanitary towels or tampons used, but one cannot record these two forms of protection as equal, and some patients use one or the other at different times, or even both when bleeding is heavy. Cooperation was poor and we soon abandoned the method as unworkable. Hallberg's work showed that women are unable to define their menstrual loss in absolute terms. Nevertheless we ask patients to summarise their total bleeding as heavy, moderate or light. This seems paradoxical, but the individual subject should be able to recognise changes in her total menstrual loss, even though the terms that she uses mean nothing on any absolute scale. We can then compare the percentage of women who describe their bleeding as heavy, moderate or light in each cycle and see what overall effect the pill is having.

How is the bleeding pattern analysed? A pill has been given that is designed to produce an artificial withdrawal bleed at regular intervals of twentyeight days and to suppress natural menstruation completely. It may appear a simple matter to describe the frequency and duration of unwanted bleeding, that is bleeding occurring while the tablets are being taken. We will call it 'breakthrough bleeding' if it requires sanitary protection, and 'spotting' if it does not.

But problems arise. Is it right to call bleeding 'breakthrough bleeding' at the beginning of a course of tablets, even if it is a continuation of withdrawal bleeding? If it is considered part of withdrawal bleeding, after how many days of the next course ought we to start describing it as breakthrough bleeding? What if there has been no withdrawal bleeding at the proper time, but bleeding of significant length and amount occurs at the beginning of the next course? Is it correct to include that episode in 'withdrawal bleeding', perhaps as a subcategory of 'delayed withdrawal bleeding'?

Similarly, if there is a single episode of bleeding, but it starts a day or two before the last pill, should that be ignored in the analysis of breakthrough bleeding? When withdrawal bleeding does not occur should this always be described as 'amenorrhoea', or should this term not be used when there has been breakthrough bleeding during the previous course of tablets? Is it preferable not to use the misleading term 'amenorrhoea' at all when dealing with these artificial cycles, but simply to report long cycles when one or more withdrawal bleeds have been missed? There are many such questions of interpretation that confront the investigator and for which consistent rules have to be devised. No two investigators have formulated identical sets of rules, and comparison of analysis carried out by different investigators can therefore be grossly misleading. The worst solution is to leave the interpretation to the individual trialist in a multicentre trial and to allow him to report his interpretation of the data.

My experience has shown that the analysis must be carried out by no more than one or two people. They must have a written set of rules to which they can refer, and they must work directly from the patient's diary cards. I have described elsewhere a system of analysis that yields a reasonable impression of the data (Bye, 1976). It is just one of several satisfactory systems. A universal system is needed, and until such a system is agreed, comparison of the bleeding patterns produced by different oral contraceptives will be difficult, unless the various analyses were carried out by the same workers. An entirely different system is required for oral contraceptives such as the progestogen only pill, which does not impose artificial cycles. Then the impossible task of classifying bleeding episodes as menstrual or intermenstrual is not attempted (Rodriguez, Faundes-Latham & Atkinson, 1976).

Practical and statistical problems make significant comparisons of efficacy between one oral contraceptive and another impossible. Yet nearly all the trials still seem to have as their overriding objective the amassing of an impressive looking total of cycles. This imposes limitations on trial design which prevent a successful study of what, in the absence of precise information about efficacy, should in fact be the main object of the trial: That is the assessment of side effects.

### Concurrent symptoms

What people insist on calling side effects, can only be properly called 'concurrent symptoms' in the absence of placebo controls. Their variation is so great even between different trials of the same pill, as to make useless any comparison between most previous trials. Variability can be reduced by standardising the collection of  information about symptoms. Much effort has been expended in recent years by a working party (of which I am a member, and which contains representatives of all the other major pill manufacturers) to design a standard procedure for uncontrolled trials (1974). Do not subject either the women in your trial or the overworked investigators to a wearisome and largely meaningless rigmarole of questions. Many of the questionnaires used in pill trials have been taken from the routine used in family planning clinics. This in turn incorporates many questions transferred uncritically from the routine used in obstetrical and gynaecological clinics. The working party found a tremendous variation between trial protocols, and decided to subject every question that anyone asked to three tests. One: Would the answer to the question be relevant to the appraisal of the pill? Two: Could the answers to the question be reasonably accurate? Three: Could such answers be analysed statistically? A large number of widely used questions failed to pass one or other of these tests. We were left with a modest list of questions that we were sure would be relevant and useful. We paid particular attention to the technique for eliciting symptoms. We rejected questions about a long list of possible side effects, since the procedure tends to evoke too many false positives and to give a distorted picture by emphasising the listed items as compared with those not listed. We also rejected a simple enquiry, such as 'Have you had any problems?', because significant symptoms may emerge by chance at the end of the interview after a general enquiry has failed to elicit them. We produced a list of seven specific questions directed to systems or functions, and a final general question to pick up anything else. We devised a lengthy glossary to standardise the coding of the many different terms that subjects might use to describe their symptoms. A standardised scheme such as this would be a great advantage.

### The problem of controls

Placebo controls are essential to show the true incidence of subjective side effects. It is a problem to provide them. Firstly, it is not easy to find large numbers of subjects for pill trials. With a new form of therapy, one may be offering hope to patients who are willing to clutch at straws, but pill users are healthy women with little motivation to take part in a trial, especially since the pill is now available free. The provision of free contraception during the trial is no longer an incentive. The total of cycles on the new pill must be halved if all available patients are divided equally between the new pill and a control product. Alternatively, there is the problem of spending twice as much on what is already a fairly expensive exercise. Secondly, subjects for pill trials are usually recruited from among women asking for oral contraception. It is wrong to give a placebo to any of them without providing genuine contraception at the same time. This is both difficult to arrange and presents problems in preserving the double blind technique. Only Goldzieher et al. (1971) have undertaken the difficult task of double blind trial against placebo by using a chemical spermicide with the placebo (and with some of the active pills to preserve 'blindness'). Goldzieher preserved his patients' 'blindness' by telling them that they must use the spermicide for the first few months until it was known that they were taking an effective pill. He does not seem to have told them a placebo was to be included. This is probably justifiable, provided that sufficient stress is placed on the need for taking seriously the use of the additional contraceptive.

For between pill comparisons, a double blind crossover can be used. This has been done by Nilsson & Sölvell (1976) with four pills taken in randomised order, with one cycle for each pill, repeating the same order in cycles five to eight and nine to twelve. This was a good design, which tended to cancel out the effects of habituation.

Space does not permit me to discuss in detail other aspects of limited value that are studied in pill trials. Gonadotrophins and sex hormones will not enable us to predict anything about post-pill amenorrhoea. They will indicate when ovulation occurs, but we know from work on the progestogen-only minipill that the inhibition of ovulation is not essential to hormonal contraception. A study of the cervical mucus alone does not indicate what contraceptive effects the pill has, although in the post-coital test it may do so. A study of endometrial biopsies is unhelpful, since we have no idea what contribution endometrial changes make to the overall effectiveness of oral contraceptives. Measurement of coagulation and anticoagulation factors and plasma lipids do not indicate the risk of thrombosis. Glucose tolerance tests tell us nothing about morbidity.

My chief reason for mentioning these tests is to point out that we accept that they can be done only on small groups of subjects. The same individual approach should be adopted to the traditional features of a clinical trial of an oral contraceptive. We should cease pursuing the will - o'-the-wisp of efficacy. We should concentrate on well designed double blind trials that will give reliable information, not only about cycle-control but also about weight gain, depression, loss of libido and other so-called side-effects, which even after many years of oral contraception are still questionable, or at least unquantifiable. Metabolic studies should be done because, if two pills cause different degrees of metabolic disturbance, the one that causes the lesser disturbance is surely the less likely to cause morbidity.

Well controlled clinical trials of oral contraceptives cannot encompass the statistical evaluation of rare events, such as pregnancy and thromboembolism. Such evaluation must await retrospective case control studies, or extremely large prospective studies, such as that of the Royal College of General Practitioners. These are outside the scope of this discussion. No study on such a scale will be undertaken until a product has undergone normal clinical evaluation and has shown itself to be suitable for wide spread use.

If we want to carry out truly scientific trials of oral contraceptives, we must identify the attainable objectives and pursue them singlemindedly.

REFERENCES

Bye, P. (1976) Analysis of a multi-centre trial of a new low-dose oral contraceptive in
    Great Britain, *Acta Obstetricia et Gynecologica Scandinavica,* Supplement **54**, 61 - 66

Chiazze, L. Jr., Brayer, F.T., Macisco, J.J. Jr., Parker, M.P. & Duffy, B.N. (1968)
    The length and variability of the human menstrual cycle. *The Journal of the
    American Medical Association,* **203**, 377.

Goldzieher, J.W., Moses, L.E., Averkin, E., Scheel, C, & Taber, B.Z. (1971) A placebo
    controlled double blind crossover investigation of the side effects attributed to
    oral contraceptives. *Fertility and Sterility,* **22**, 9: 609.

Hallberg, L., Hogdahl, A.M., Nilsson, L. & Rybo, G. (1966) Menstrual blood loss -
    a population study, *Acta Obstetricia et Gynecologica Scandinavica,* **45**, 320.

Hines, D.C. & Goldzieher, J.W. (1969) Clinical investigation: A guide to its evaluation.
    *American Journal of Obstetrics and Gynecology.* **105**, 450.

Nilsson, L. & Sölvell, L. (1967) Clinical studies on oral contraceptives - a randomized,
    doubleblind crossover study of 4 different preparations (Anovlar mite, Lyndiol mite,
    Ovulen and Volidan), *Acta Obstetricia et Gynecologica Scandinavica,* Vol. XLVI,
    Suppl. 8, 3 - 31.

Rodriguez, G., Faundes-Latham, A. & Atkinson, L.E. (1976) An approach to the
    analysis of menstrual patterns in the critical evaluation of contraceptives. *Studies
    in Family Planning,* Vol. 7, No. 2, 42 - 51.

The Control of Oral Contraceptive Clinical Trials, A Working Party Report (1974)
    The Family Planning Research Unit, University of Exeter.

# 19. Antidepressant and Anxiolytic Trials

G. BEAUMONT

Clinical trials of anxiolytic and antidepressant drugs require essentially the same approach as that required for any form of therapeutic investigation. As in all studies planning and adequate preparation are essential. The haphazard collection of data in the hope that their subsequent analysis will produce something of interest and worth is invariably of little value. The cornerstone of a good clinical trial is the trial protocol, the preparation of which should be as meticulous as possible.

It is useful to consider the preparation of the protocol under the following sub-headings:

Aim
Population
Trial design
Criteria for admission
Exclusions
Methodology
Indices for measuring change
Dose
Side effects
Other drugs
'Drop outs', withdrawals
Dispensing arrangements
Statistics

## Aim

A good clinical trial should always begin with a declaration of intent, and what it is hoped the trial will achieve. There is a great temptation to try to get as much 'mileage' out of a clinical trial as possible and collect a mass of data about every conceivable aspect of the subject under study. Such an approach not infrequently spells disaster for a clinical study. 'Keep it simple' is a good principle to bear in mind. It is better to have limited objectives which can be achieved than complex ones which prove impossible. Thus in clinical trials of antidepressants or anxiolytics the objective might be to assess the clinical efficacy of a trial compound as compared with placebo therapy or treatment with a reference compound. Coupled with this will usually be an evaluation of tolerance. Nowadays there is an increasing tendency, due to the advent of the appropriate technology, to relate both efficacy and tolerance to blood levels of the drug being administered. Differing dose levels or regimes of the same compound may be compared.

## Population

The protocol should state what patients are to be admitted to the study. Are both sexes to be included? What is the age limit? Children will be excluded unless the trial is expressly designed to study effects in the young. The behaviour of drugs in the elderly both clinically and metabolically differs frequently from that in younger patients. This must be borne in mind when selecting an age range.

An increasing number of clinical trials of antidepressant and anxiolytic compounds are now being performed in general practice. There are good reasons for this development. The advantages of conducting such trials in hospital either on in or out patients are that diagnosis is likely to be more accurate; more varied facilities exist for assessment and in general, much more time is available for such procedures. However, there are many disadvantages. Today most depressed or anxious patients are treated by their general practitioners at first. It is only when they fail to respond or some other factor arises that they are referred to a psychiatric clinic. Thus the hospital population is not typical but selected. Moreover, an already drug-contaminated population makes many studies, especially of blood levels, difficult to perform. The hospital population tends to be overweighted with patients with social or personality problems. These frequently drive the general practitioner to seek the help of his specialist colleagues and the attendant ancillary services. In practice hospital trials take a long time to recruit suitable patients. Experience with trials of antidepressant compounds has shown that an admission rate of about thirty new patients a year is usual. This means that an adequate clinical trial is a lengthy procedure.

By contrast the general practitioner (G.P.) sees a plentiful supply of previously untreated and relatively uncomplicated patients suffering from depression or anxiety. Not all patients seen by the general practitioner are really depressed or anxious in the sense of having a true clinical disorder. They may have a depressive reaction rather than a true depressive illness. They may be somewhat inadequate people overstressed rather than sufferers from a pathological anxiety state. This difference must be resolved in drawing up the admission criteria. It may also be argued that the G.P. does not have sufficient time for adequate assessment and diagnosis. Nevertheless, the advantages of conducting such research in general practice outweigh its disadvantages. If it is desirable to recruit large numbers of patients in a relatively short time, the multicentre approach must be considered. This requires considerable effort to ensure uniformity in the application of admission criteria and in assessment.

## Trial design

Clinical trials of anxiolytics and antidepressants may be uncontrolled or controlled. In general, controlled studies carry greater conviction. If the control therapy is another drug or placebo the double blind approach is usually possible and desirable. If the comparison is to be made with some other type of therapy, such as electroconvulsive therapy, psychotherapy or behaviour therapy, the comparison must be open. Even the employment of independent assessors is fraught with difficulties. Usually the clinical trial of an anxiolytic or antidepressant compound is a double blind controlled comparison with either a reference drug or a placebo. The use of placebo in such studies, particularly if conducted on outpatients or general practice patients, is contentious because of the risk of overdosage and suicide. This is as much an ethical and medicolegal problem as it is clinical.

Comparative trials may be performed between patients or within patients. Between patient trials require some attempt at matching treatment groups. This is best achieved by stratification. Stratification factors should be selected on statistical grounds and prognostic significance, such as sex, age, severity and duration of illness. In general, limit the number of stratification factors to four, or at the most five. Contrary to a widespread misconception, it is not necessary to recruit the same number of patients to each stratification subgroup.

Within patient comparative studies have limited value. It is difficult to account for 'carry over' effects clinically and in tissue drug levels. The patient's condition at the start of two respective treatment periods is rarely comparable. The necessity to introduce 'wash out' periods between treatments creates management problems. Probably the only use for within patient methods is in the study of chronic anxiety states. Here sequential analysis could be used. This method might also be utilised with matched pairs. Usually pair matching is difficult: A between patients study employing stratification factors is more desirable and practical.

I have already referred to the single centre or multicentre approach. The first usually takes longer to recruit an adequate number of patients but provides greater uniformity in selection and assessment. Multicentre studies provide an opportunity to recruit large numbers of patients quickly but have the disadvantage of variable standards.

## Criteria for admission

The trial protocol should lay down as precisely as possible the clinical basis on which patients are to be selected and admitted to a clinical trial. There are no universally agreed criteria for either depression or anxiety. Therefore it is important that an investigator should define his own standards and communicate clearly to others his basis for selection. Controversy still surrounds the diagnosis of depression, particularly regarding the endogenous and reactive differentiation of depression and the unitary concept. It may be more appropriate to describe admission criteria on the basis of the presence or absence of certain target symptoms.

Similar problems are posed by anxiety. The distinction between normal and abnormal anxiety is not easy. In addition it may be necessary to distinguish between psychic and somatic anxiety and between acute and chronic conditions. The study may be further complicated if the anxiety accompanies some other condition such as phobic state.

It is impossible at present to lay down clear and rigid criteria for admission to antidepressant and anxiolytic trials, since there are not universally accepted standards. Therefore it might be better to describe target symptoms rather than define syndromes.

## Exclusions

It is as important for the trial protocol to clearly indicate which patients are to be excluded as it is to describe those that are to be included. Exclusion must be justified. If the drug has unwanted pharmacological effects, it would be prudent to exclude patients with certain other diseases. Thus patients with glaucoma or prostatism might be excluded from a trial of an antidepressant, and patients with liver disease would be excluded from trial of a drug with possible hepatotoxicity. Whatever the results of teratology, it is wise to exclude all pregnant patients unless the trial is specifically concerned with disorders of pregnancy. For reasons already stated children will be excluded from general studies. The elderly may be excluded or special provision made for them.

Depression and anxiety often complicate other psychiatric disorders. This makes evaluation difficult. If a straight assessment of antidepressive or anxiolytic effect is required it is best to exclude patients with such conditions as schizophrenia.

Often patients are taking other drugs for unrelated conditions. If these must be continued on ethical grounds then the possibility of interaction must be considered. If this is thought likely or probable such patients must be excluded from the trial. Occasionally previous therapy must be considered. For instance, patients previously treated with a monoamine oxidase inhibitor should not be treated with a tricyclic antidepressant within fourteen days. Whether treatments interact or not, patients with unrelated progressive disease are best excluded from the straight assessment. A special trial may be conducted for such subjects.

### Methodology

A section of the protocol should define the procedure for the study. It describes the data to be collected at the outset and during the conduct of the trial. These will include details of patients' sex, age, history of the present condition, history of previous attacks, the therapy given and the response obtained, the presence of other disease and the use of other drugs. The possible list of initial data is limitless. You should consider whether this collection of data is useful in the final analysis, otherwise time is wasted. The assessment programme should be defined. How long will the trial last and what will be the frequency of assessment? Rapid onset of action may be important. The assessment programme should be so constructed as to discern the earliest signs of effect. Special details should be clarified. For instance, if blood levels are to be measured, times and conditions of sampling and assessment should be standardised. Every patient in the trial must be treated in a similar way. The methodology section should ensure that this is so.

### Indices for assessment change

The measuring instrument used is crucial to any clinical trial. There are special problems in measuring change in depression and anxiety since the assessment can only be made subjectively. Assessments may be made by physicians, by patients themselves, by relatives, nurses or other ancillary workers. When choosing a measuring instrument, distinguish between those devices which are purely diagnostic and those which clearly demonstrate symptomatic change. Many methods of assessment used in depression or anxiety are diagnostic tools. Once the diagnosis is made they are not sufficiently sensitive to pick up change. On the other hand there are measuring devices which depend on the diagnosis having been made first. These are then sufficiently sensitive to indicate changes in symptom severity. In general such devices should be selected for use in clinical trials of anxiolytics and antidepressants. When using new clinical measuring tools, make sure they are valid and reliable.

Rating scales are the assessments most widely used by physicians. Well known examples are the Hamilton Scale for Depression and the Hamilton Scale for Anxiety.

Patient assessments may be similar but questionnaires or linear and visual analogue scales are more usual. Examples are the Beck Depression Inventory or the Wakefield Scale for Depression and the Taylor Manifest Anxiety Scale for anxiety. The visual analogue scale has a ten centimetre line at the ends of which are two extreme opposite symptomatic experiences. The patient rates his current condition between the two extremes. Rating scales have been developed for use by relatives, nurses and other ancillary workers. Global assessment as better, the same or worse, made either by the patient or the physician, has been found to be as reliable as any other means of assessing change.

## Dose

The protocol must lay down the dose of drug to be used whether fixed or variable. Fixed dosage studies are more easily analysed statistically. However, they only provide information about what happens at that dose and leave many management problems unanswered. Variable dosage resembles the real clinical situation more closely but creates analytical difficulties. The choice of the comparable dose of a reference drug is also difficult. It must be a dose that is assumed to be equipotent. When altered formulations and presentations of drugs are used to permit matching in blind trials, bioavailability must be comparable to standard preparations. Otherwise the results obtained may be quite misleading.

The question of dosage has been confused by recent discoveries about the blood levels of antidepressant and anxiolytic drugs. There is wide individual variation following a standard dose. It is now, therefore, questionable whether the dose should be fixed or whether the aim should be to achieve optimal blood levels. The concept of individually adjusted dose is now being considered in the design of clinical trials.

The dose regime also should be defined. Single dose therapy (at night) of antidepressants now enjoys some popularity. The patient's cooperation must be considered when choosing the dose and particularly the dose regime. One of the biggest problems in trials is the failure of patients to take their medication correctly. Various estimates of patient compliance have been made. It has been suggested that up to 40 per cent of patients being treated with psychotropic drugs do not take them properly. Moreover, the more frequent the dosage, the greater is the risk of the patient not complying. Attempts have been made to check on patient compliance. Urinary markers, such as riboflavin and tablet counts have been used. None have proved entirely satisfactory. Now that blood levels of some psychotropic drugs can be measured, sampling will at least show whether the patient has taken and absorbed any of the drug or not.

## Side effects

A standard procedure should be defined in the protocol for the assessment of side effects and for routine pathological, haematological or biochemical tests. The manner of eliciting side effects from patients should be described and repeated at each assessment. With antidepressant and anxiolytic drugs it is preferable to rely on volunteered or observed side effects. The volunteered effects should be recorded in response to some standard question.

It is most important to identify any symptoms which might subsequently be regarded as side effects before treatment has commenced. Many of the side effects of antidepressant and anxiolytic drugs are also symptoms of the conditions they are intended to treat. Thus, unless baseline information is collected, results obtained during a clinical trial may be quite misleading. It has been shown that many socalled drug-induced side effects are, in fact, present before therapy commences.

### Other drugs

The protocol must make provision for patients taking other drugs being admitted to the study. The importance of possible drug interactions is being increasingly realised. Drugs may interact in a variety of ways. One may interfere with absorption of another; one drug may induce enzymes and alter metabolism; they may compete for protein binding sites; one may alter the metabolism of another thus altering blood levels and enhancing or reducing clinical response or side effects. Drugs may also compete with each other pharmacologically and disturb the control of symptoms as a result of simultaneous administration. It is, therefore, extremely important that potential drug interactions should be considered if additional medication is allowed during the clinical trial. Interactions with oral contraceptives are possible and there is some evidence to suggest that smoking habits may influence the metabolism of psychotropic drugs.

For example, there are problems when giving tricyclic antidepressants to patients on adrenergic blocking drugs for the treatment of hypertension. These remarks concern the use of prescribed drugs. Little is known about possible interactions with self medication.

### Dropouts and withdrawals

Some patients are inevitably withdrawn from, or drop out of, a clinical trial. It is important to record the reasons and time of withdrawal from the study. In the analysis of the trial, a decision must be made as to whether these reasons for dropout are drug related or not. Are they due to side effects or not? They may be disease related, the patient deteriorating or getting better and not wishing to remain in the trial. Although difficult to handle statistically, dropouts and withdrawals can provide valuable clinical information.

### Dispensing arrangements

The protocol should specify the dispensing arrangements. In hospital these should be handled by the hospital pharmacy. Drugs may, if necessary, be dispensed from bulk. Special prescription forms will be required, especially if stratification factors are used. Prepared containers will be required in general practice. This creates a problem which may be important in the treatment of anxiety and depressive states since these are known to have a high placebo response rate. The patient is, in fact, being given a 'special pill' rather than an EC10. This may influence the patient's attitude to treatment.

There is a risk of overdose or suicide in antidepressant or anxiolytic trials. Therefore proper arrangements must be made for emergency breaking of the individual code. This must not destroy the blindness of the rest of the study. The problem is resolved in hospital if the pharmacist keeps the code. In general practice individual numbered envelopes should be used to allow the code to be broken for a single patient.

Many patients may be required to continue the trial drug after the end of the trial. This continuation therapy must be provided in such a manner as to preserve the secrecy of the treatment schedule.

## Statistics

As with all clinical trials statistical advice should be sought when planning the trial. The investigator's most difficult problem is knowing how many patients will be required for any particular study. The number of patients required will depend on the order of differences he would like to show. This has been discussed in detail in Chapter 9.

There are special problems when planning clinical trials of antidepressant and anxiolytic drugs. Nevertheless the same principles apply to trials of these drugs as to any other trial. Trials of antidepressant and anxiolytic drugs have been considered in this chapter on the basis of thirteen sections. These should form an integral part of any clinical trial protocol.

# 20. Trials of Anti-rheumatic Drugs

E. C. HUSKISSON

Trials of anti-rheumatic drugs must be designed according to the properties of the drug to be tested. The properties of a new drug can sometimes be predicted from animal studies or from preliminary clinical work: more often, it is necessary to design a programme of trials to document activity or lack of activity of different types and also demonstrate toxicity of various types. The principle consideration which determines the design of trial required is the time course of the action of the drug. The expected action determines the type of patient to be treated and the measurements which will be made.

Rheumatoid arthritis is a common disease, and being characterised by both pain and inflammation, provides an ideal test situation for anti-rheumatic drugs. This chapter will therefore deal mainly with rheumatoid arthritis. Important variations in design of trials and measurements to be made in other diseases will also be discussed.

## Classification and chronopharmacology of drugs used for rheumatoid arthritis

Anti-rheumatic drugs have been produced in large numbers in recent years and it is therefore particularly important that they should be classified. The clinical classification shown in Table 20.1 was suggested by Huskisson (1974a). Propionic acid derivatives were classed as 'analgesics with minor anti-inflammatory activity', which is appropriate to ibuprofen but less so to the more active members of the group. It therefore seems more suitable to class them as 'propionic acid derivatives and similar compounds'. It is important to distinguish these from the traditional anti-inflammatory drugs like aspirin.

The chronopharmacology of these drugs deserves emphasis. The time taken for the maximal effect of a drug to develop is a major factor in the design of a trial. For example, the maximal effect of simple analgesics occurs 2 or 3 hours after administration. Measurement of pain relief at this time will readily detect the activity of a drug like paracetamol but measurement at another time, for example after a week of regular dosing, may not (Huskisson, 1974b). D-penicillamine takes 4 to 6 months to exert its maximal effect: a time course of this type is characteristic of such drugs and is useful confirmation of these properties. Side effects also occur at characteristic times; for example, loss of taste in patients receiving D-penicillamine usually develops at about the sixth week of treatment while proteinuria occurs between the fourth and eighteenth months. This will clearly influence the duration of a trial designed to determine the incidence of such toxic effects in a new drug.

188

Table 20.1  Classification of anti-rheumatic drugs

| | |
|---|---|
| Simple analgesics | Paracetamol, aspirin (small doses), codeine, dihydrocodeine, dextropropoxyphene and combinations of these. |
| Analgesic anti-inflammatory drugs<br>    Propionic acid derivatives and<br>    compounds with similar activity | Propionic acid derivatives: fenoprofen, ketoprofen, ibuprofen, naproxen |
| | Acetic acid derivatives: Alclofenac |
| | Fenamates: flufenamic acid, mefenamic acid |
| Aspirin and compounds with<br>    similar activity | Aspirin (large doses), indomethacin, phenylbutazone, oxyphenbutazone |
| Pure anti-inflammatory drugs | Corticosteroids and ACTH |
| Drugs with a specific action in<br>rheumatoid arthritis | Penicillamine, gold, chloroquine, immunosuppressives, levamisole |

Simple analgesics relieve pain without any effect on inflammation; they act within 30 minutes and reach a peak after 2 to 3 hours. The action declines thereafter and disappears within a few hours. A subsequent dose has exactly the same effect and regular dosing does not increase the activity. Anti-inflammatory drugs also relieve pain but when given regularly, there is a gradual increase in their effect over the course of a few days. Relief of pain is accompanied by improvement in some manifestations of inflammation such as stiffness and swelling. Drugs with a specific action in rheumatoid arthritis have no immediate effect but regular administration produces a gradual amelioration of symptoms and signs of the disease over the course of a few months. This is accompanied by improvement in extra- articular manifestations of the disease such as nodules and reduction in the titre of rheumatoid factor, E.S.R. and immunoglobulins.

## Propionic acid derivatives and variations in responsiveness

The difference in action between propionic acid derivatives and drugs like aspirin is subtle but important. There is a very obvious difference in the incidence of side effects. Propionic acid derivatives do not reduce proximal interphalangeal joint circumference in short-term trials (with treatment periods of 1 or 2 weeks) though they probably do eventually. Reduction in joint swelling was regarded as the hallmark of anti-inflammatory action (characteristic of aspirin, indomethacin and phenylbutazone) and led to the suggestion that these drugs were not anti-inflammatory. However the time course of their action is similar to that of the anti-inflammatory drugs and they produce improvement in morning stiffness, a characteristic of inflammatory arthropathies (which seems to have been overlooked by Celsus and Galen when they described the cardinal signs of inflammation). It is an indication of the inadequacy of existing methods that we are not able to document this anti-inflammatory effect in a more satisfactory way.

A striking variation in responsiveness to propionic acid derivatives has recently been demonstrated (Huskisson et al., 1976). It is clear that each of these drugs is effective in only a proportion of the population. This has enormous implications in clinical trials. It would be easy to select a group of patients who would not respond to one of these drugs and another which would respond very well. It is clearly necessary to study larger numbers of patients than has been usual in comparative trials of drugs of this type. Some variation exists in responses to all drugs; for example an unpredictable 20 per cent of patients with rheumatoid arthritis fail to respond to D-penicillamine. With more drugs available today, it is the non-responders who attend clinics most frequently and complain most loudly. One must avoid including a majority of such patients in trials of new drugs.

### Anti-rheumatic drug trial programme

A programme suitable for complete evaluation of a new drug with potential activity for rheumatic diseases is shown in Table 20.2. Some modification of the programme will be made on the basis of animal pharmacology, studies in volunteers and pilot trials in patients.

*Trials of simple analgesics* (Huskisson, 1974b)

*Design.* Simple analgesics are used in single doses taken on demand and should be tested in this way. An ideal design is a multiple crossover trial in which the unknown drug is compared with a placebo and a standard active control, such as aspirin or paracetamol. It seems that better results are obtained when each compound is given more than once; three times has been found to give good results. Comparison of the treatments in pairs allows patients to express preferences but these are less sensitive in showing effectiveness than pain relief scores. Order of treatment should be random-ised and balanced and only one trial dose per day should be given to avoid possible carry-over effects.

*Patients.* Patients must have chronic pain of sufficient severity to require adminis-tration of analgesics at least once each day. Experience suggests that 24 patients are sufficient to document the effects of drugs like paracetamol and aspirin.

*Drugs.* The test drugs should be identical since colour and appearance may influence response. Other therapy may be continued provided that it remains unchanged through-out the study and that it does not include any of the test drugs.

*Measurements.* Pain relief is the only useful measurement. It should be measured hourly for six hours after administration of test drugs using either a simple descriptive scale (non, slight, moderate and complete relief of pain) or a visual analogue scale (Huskisson, 1974c). The use of a pain relief scale, rather than a scale of pain severity, eliminates the effect of variation in initial pain score on response.

*Trials of anti-inflammatory drugs*

*Design.* Most anti-inflammatory drugs are fully effective within a few days and their effects wear off within a similar time. It is therefore possible to use a crossover design,

Table 20.2  A programme of clinical trials for a potential anti-rheumatic drug

| Stage | Type of action demonstrated | Design of study | Measurements |
|---|---|---|---|
| 1 | Analgesic | Single dose multiple crossover | Pain relief |
| 2 | Anti-inflammatory | Three-way crossover with one or two week treatment periods | Pain<br><br>Duration of morning stiffness<br><br>Articular index<br><br>Grip strength<br><br>Preference<br><br>Analgesic requirements<br><br>Proximal interphalangeal joint circumference |
| 3 | Toxicity and specific activity in rheumatoid arthritis | Group comparative study lasting at least six months | As for anti-inflammatory plus:<br><br>E.S.R.<br><br>Rheumatoid factor titre<br><br>Immunoglobulins<br><br>Technetium Index<br><br>Side effects<br><br>Haematology, biochemistry, urinalysis and specific toxicity tests |
| 4 | Confirmatory trials, trials in conditions other than rheumatoid arthritis and comparative trials using different reference drugs | Various depending on effects to be demonstrated | Various depending on effects to be demonstrated |
| 5 | Uncommon side effects | Monitored release | Side effects<br><br>Haematology etc. as appropriate |

giving each drug for one week and comparing unknown, placebo and a standard active compound. With the variability in responsiveness of patients, it is particularly important to include an active compound as well as placebo. Comparison of standard active compound and placebo shows whether the patients were capable of response, comparison of unknown and placebo shows whether the unknown was effective and comparison of unknown and standard active drug shows how effective it was. The order of treatment should be randomised and balanced. Some compounds with a long half life take more than one week to work and in this circumstance, the period of treatment

must be prolonged or crossover methodology abandoned in favour of a group comparative study. It is unkind and usually unnecessary to give placebo for longer than one week.

*Patients.*   Experience suggests that 12 to 18 patients with active disease are sufficient
to show that a drug like aspirin is superior to placebo, but this is only a crude screening
test of effectiveness. Much larger numbers of patients are required to obtain information
about variability and frequency of response but such information can be obtained at
a later stage. Active disease is a term which clinicians understand, but which is difficult
to define.

*Drugs.*   Such trials should be double blind. No other anti-inflammatory therapy should
be allowed during the trial but patients on a small dose of steroid are often included
provided that they have active disease and that the dose of steroid has been constant
for a few months. The same applies to patients who have been receiving gold, penicillamine and other specific agents. The inclusion of patients on these other types of
drugs does not interfere with the demonstration of effectiveness of the test compound.
Simple analgesics are allowed: the requirement is measured by returned tablet counting
and used as a measure of effectiveness. Choice of a control compound is difficult.
Aspirin has been widely used for this purpose but is now being supplanted in general
use by propionic acid derivatives. One of the more effective of these such as fenoprofen
or naproxen can therefore be used as an alternative.

*Measurements.*   Conventional measurements are shown in Table 20.2. These should be
made at the end of each treatment period by the same observer and at the same time
of day on each occasion. The principle of such trials is that the patients equilibrate on
each treatment and that their equilibrium state on each is compared. It is therefore an
error to measure changes which occur during a treatment period and for the same reason
it is better to measure the severity of pain rather than pain relief. A visual analogue
scale is convenient for this purpose. Pain and preference have proved to be the most
reliable tests in such trials. The duration of morning stiffness must be included as a
measure of anti-inflammatory potency. Proximal interphalangeal joint circumference
(Boardman and Hart, 1967) should also be included though it is not reduced in such
trials by propionic acid derivatives. Many patients with rheumatoid arthritis are not
capable of showing a reduction in joint swelling even with aspirin and similar drugs.
Grip strength and articular index are useful additions; the latter is available in simple
form as described by Ritchie *et al.* (1968). Thermography and technetium counting
have not yet been shown to be useful measures of anti-inflammatory therapy.

### Long-term trials

Long term treatment, at least six months, is required to document the side effects
and toxicity of a compound and to determine whether it has a specific effect on
rheumatoid arthritis. These two aims can conveniently be combined in the same trial.

*Design.*   Group-comparative trials are usually preferred for this type of trial though
crossovers with four month treatment periods have been successfully completed. It is
a pity to stop treatment even after six months if good progress has been made on one
drug: this requires parallel groups.

*Patients.* For trials of penicillamine-like drugs, patients should be chosen in whom such treatment is indicated: Those with persistently active disease despite optimal anti-inflammatory therapy and those showing progression either with developing deformities or radiological deterioration. Twelve patients in each group are sufficient to show the effectiveness of penicillamine over a control group on anti-inflammatory terhapy. At least 30 patients in each group are required in trials designed to show the incidence of side effects or to compare two active drugs.

*Drugs.* Long-term trials of this type need not be double blind, especially when assessments are made by an independant observer. In this circumstance, side effects must be collected independantly of data on effectiveness in order that characteristic symptoms do not unblind the observer. Readily identifiable medication which patients may already have received should not be used. In trials of penicillamine-like drugs, anti-inflammatory therapy must be continued since the action of these drugs is slow. It is usual to establish an optimal treatment regime before the first assessment. Dosage may then be reduced and the requirements used as a measure of effectiveness. Choice of a control drug will depend on the aims of the trial; in long term trials of anti-inflammatory agents, another anti-inflammatory drug such as a propionic acid derivative should be used; in trials of drugs with a specific action in rheumatoid arthritis, one group may receive anti-inflammatory therapy only or penicillamine may be used as a control substance.

*Measurements.* Measurements to be made in long-term trials are shown in Table 20.2. Drugs like penicillamine can be identified by their effects on extra-articular features of the disease. It is useful to make a count of elbow nodules and to document the presence of other extra articular features. Measurement of E.S.R. rheumatoid factor titre and immunoglobulins should be made before treatment and after 3 and 6 months. Reduction in technetium index has been shown to be produced by drugs of this type but not by anti-inflammatory drugs.

Measurement of the side effects of drugs is notoriously difficult. Patients should be seen at regular intervals and the presence of side effects elicited by a standard question such as 'Has the treatment upset you in any way?' The use of a check list interferes with the collection of side effects (Huskisson and Wojtulewski, 1974).

### Further trials

These three trials will document the analgesic, anti-inflammatory and specific activity and toxicity of most drugs in rheumatoid arthritis. The next phase of the investigation should include similar trials in conditions other than rheumatoid arthritis, such as osteoarthritis, and in other conditions in which the drug might be indicated; and comparative trials to compare the properties of the new drug with the most widely used drugs already in use.

Formal toxicity trials detect only the most frequent side effects. The incidence of unwanted effects should be carefully observed in a much larger group of patients. This is best achieved by monitored release in specific centres.

### Trials in conditions other than rheumatoid arthritis

Similar principles apply to trials in other rheumatic diseases. Analgesic and anti-inflammatory studies can be carried out in osteoarthritis but the only useful measurements which can be made are pain, preference and stiffness after inactivity. Similar trials in ankylosing spondylitis require measurement of pain, preference and range of spinal movement.

The natural history of the condition must also be considered. Trials in acute gout or the various types of soft tissue rheumatism must be designed in the knowledge that these conditions resolve spontaneously. Group comparative trials must therefore be used. In trials of specific therapy for gout, with drugs like allopurinal, measurement of serum uric acid and the number of attacks of gout are required.

## REFERENCES

Boardman, P.L. & Hart, F.D. (1967) *British Medical Journal,* **4**, 264 - 268.

Huskisson, E.C. (1974a) Reports of Rheumatic Diseases No. 54. Arthritis and Rheumatism Council.

Huskisson, E.C. (1974b) *British Medical Journal,* **4**, 196 - 200.

Huskisson, E.C. (1974c) *Lancet,* **2**, 1127 - 1131.

Huskisson, E.C. & Wojtulewski, J.A. (1974) *British Medical Journal,* **2**, 698 - 699.

Huskisson, E.C., Woolf, D.W., Balme, H.W., Scott, P.J. & Franklyn, S. (1976) *British Medical Journal,* in press.

Ritchie, D.M., Boyle, J.A., McInnes, J.M., Jasani, M.K., Dalakos, T.G., Grieveson, P. & Buchanan, W.W. (1968) *Quarterly Journal of Medicine,* **37**, 393 - 406.

# Discussion Part 4

*Dr. C.A.P. Saxton (Pfizer):*  Professor Lawrie, I wish to make sure I have got the selection criteria right. You would accept patients with stable angina with positive exercise tests for the trial; the criteria for a positive exercise test being either 1 mm or greater depression in the ST segment lasting for two minutes, or ectopic activity.

You would exclude the six per cent with negative coronary angiograms. Presumably when indirectly assessing myocardial function by systolic time interval (STI), you would wish to see reproducible uniform STIs. Is this correct, and how do you quantify the ectopic activity?

*Professor Lawrie:*  Yes, that is right. We are worried by the occurrence of three successive extrasystoles; that is what one might describe as a 'short run' ventricular tachycardia; or if the extrasystoles are multifocal, that is, if they are of differing shape. If we see these on an electrocardiogram we stop the exercise test immediately, otherwise defibrillation might be needed.

*Dr. Saxton:*  In the absence of ST depression, would you still accept that as a positive indication for accepting the patient into the trial?

*Professor Lawrie:*  Only if I could reproduce it the next time. It is a positive end point, but I would make the proviso that if it was not reproducible then such a patient could not be used for serial testing of a new antianginal compound.

*Dr. E. Vogl (Hoechst):*  Are your requirements, including coronary angiography, only meant for the early stage of the drug's evaluation, because not all the centres used later in the evaluation have these facilities? This includes general practice. Secondly, would you enlarge on the definition of stable angina?

*Professor Lawrie:*  I think coronary angiography is mandatory for selection of cases. I showed that in our experience about six per cent of cases have normal coronary vessels. I think they are suffering from a disease process different to angina secondary to coronary artery sclerosis. Therefore at some stage you must do coronary angiography.

There are two main types of angina, stable angina and unstable angina. Stable angina is angina which we recognise by chest pain of the type described in Chapter 16, which is reproduced each time with the same degree of exercise in the same period of time and with the same end point electrocardiographically.

*Dr. H.H. Soep (Bristol-Myers):*  Would Dr. Reeves clarify the difference between bacteriological cure, relapse and reinfection. For how many weeks after stopping treatment should we follow patients after urinary tract, respiratory tract and other infections? What are your objective criteria for your evaluation? When should specimens be taken?

*Dr. Reeves:* I have most experience with urinary infections. Failure of eradication or relapse shows soon after stopping treatment. Timing may not be all that important. If the same organism appears within four weeks after stopping treatment it is probably a reinfection, whereas if it appears almost immediately after stopping treatment, then it is probably a relapse. In other words reinfection can occur at any time. It is a random event whereas the chances of a relapse becoming apparent decrease rapidly within about a week of stopping treatment in urinary infections.

*Dr. M.J. Tidd (Syntex):* Dr. Bye, I would have thought that the incidence of breakthrough bleeding, however defined, is relatively easy to determine objectively. However, when I looked at first cycle breakthrough bleeding (BTB) rates (defined in such a way that would give no problems) with the same pill but different investigators, the rates varied by tenfold. Have you found a similar spread of difference across investigators? My belief in the use of diary cards for BTB evaluation was badly shattered. Do you retain any confidence in diary cards for this purpose, or in any BTB figures, and if so why?

*Dr. Bye:* If you found a great difference when the same people analysed two sets of diary cards, then I must admit to astonishment. We have found differences, but never of that order, between different trial analyses; but only when the analyses have been carried out by other investigators who have reported their own interpretation of the bleeding pattern. I am astonished at the differences you found when you did it yourself. It is possible that you were using analysts who were not working from a closely defined set of rules. There is no problem with minor variations in the bleeding pattern. A small episode of breakthrough bleeding occurring in isolation in the middle of a course of tablets with distinct withdrawal bleeding on both sides causes no problem in interpretation. Gross irregularities, particularly in the early cycles, can give rise to widely different interpretations from the same diary cards.

*Dr. M.J. Tidd (Syntex:* We worked from very closely defined rules. We checked our data very carefully because it was in fact the rules that were programmed into a computer. The machine was working correctly at the time. There was no doubt when checking the original records that these differences in the data did exist. It surprised us as much as you. I wondered whether our results are unprecedented. Judging by your wide experience, it certainly sounds as though they are.

*Dr. M.F. Corbett (Ealing):* Dr. Huskisson, you said you need large groups. How large?

*Dr. Huskisson:* It depends what you want to show. I would have thought, just looking at the data in Chapter 20, that any comparison between one propionic acid derivative and another using anything less than about 60 patients would be meaningless. I would condemn any study with only twelve or eighteen patients. It is easy to pick twelve patients who would react in a different way.

*Dr. C.T.W. Hunter (ACF. Chemieforma, Netherlands):*  Is it not possible that if you need such large groups to show a difference, then the differences must be small?

*Dr. Huskisson:*  That is so. One could have shown the difference with smaller numbers of patients. The problem is not the size needed to show the difference but the selections of a representative group. Your point is valid. I have not worked out what number you would need to show a difference between the more effective of these compounds and the less effective. One could work it out.

*Dr. E.S. Snell (Glaxo):*  Your illustration of the blood levels is shattering. One should not dismiss that quite as quickly perhaps as you have. Would you like to say any more about the reasons, the timing of those blood samples after the dose, the duration patients had been on the dose, their clearances, absorption and so on?

*Dr. Huskisson:*  I am sorry you have asked me that question. The study was moderately unsatisfactory. Blood samples were taken at the time of assessment. We recorded the time since the last dose. The times were moderately comparable but not always identical. We have done a much more elegant study subsequently. We took responders and nonresponders to two of the drugs and compared blood levels in a formal way, one hour before and after administration. With one of the drugs there was no difference between the levels in patients taken from the two extremes of the population. So blood levels just do not account for the difference in responsiveness between these drugs. I do not know where to look next for the explanation, but it is clearly not due to a difference in blood levels. Blood levels of this sort of drug just tell you whether the patient is taking it or not.

# Index